Textbook and Colour Atlas
of the Cardiovascular System

Textbook and Colour Atlas of the Cardiovascular System

C. Thomas
G. Gebert
V. Hombach

With the assistance of
L. Deichert
H. Kalbfleisch
F. Koehler
J. Rueschoff

CHAPMAN & HALL MEDICAL
London · New York · Tokyo · Melbourne · Madras

Published by Chapman & Hall, 2–6 Boundary Row, London SE1 8HN

Chapman & Hall, 2–6 Boundary Row, London SE1 8HN, UK

Van Nostrand Reinhold Inc., 115 5th Avenue, New York NY10003, USA

Chapman & Hall Japan, Thomson Publishing Japan, Hirakawacho Nemoto Building, 7F, 1-7-11 Hirakawa-cho, Chiyoda-ku, Tokyo 102, Japan

Chapman & Hall Australia, Thomas Nelson Australia, 102 Dodds Street, South Melbourne, Victoria 3205, Australia

Chapman & Hall India, R. Seshadri, 32 Second Main Road, CIT East, Madras 600 035, India

English language edition 1992

© 1992 Chapman & Hall

Original German Language edition – *Grundlagen der Klinischen Medizin 1. Herz und Gefäße* – © 1989 F.K. Schattauer Verlagsgesellschaft mbH, Stuttgart.

Typeset in Great Britain by Keyset Composition
Printed in Great Britain at the University Press, Cambridge

ISBN 0 412 43520 9   0 442 314 84 1 (USA)

A catalogue record for this book is available from the British Library

Library of Congress Cataloging-in-Publication data available

Contents

Acknowledgements

The Publishers would like to thank Mrs Rada Ivanov for her help with the translation. Grateful thanks are also due to Professor Charles Forbes, Dr Howard McAlpine and Dr Alan Bridges at the Department of Medicine, Ninewells Hospital, Dundee, for their reading of the English text and for suggesting various modifications and additions.

Sources of illustrations

Bartels, H. and Bartels, R. (1983) *Physiologie*, Urban & Schwarzenberg: Munich, Vienna, Baltimore.

Gebert, G. (1987) *Physiologie*, Schattauer: Stuttgart, New York.

Gross, R. and Schoelmerich, P. (Eds) (1982) *Lehrbuch der Inneren Medizin*, 6th edition, Schattauer: Stuttgart, New York.

Hombach, V. (Ed.) (1984) *Kardiologie. Die koronare Herzkrankheit*. H. H. Hilger: *Die nicht invasive Diagnostik der koronaren Herzkrankheit*. Schattauer: Stuttgart, New York.

Koehler, F. (1981) 'Postmortale Koronarangiographie', *Int. Welt*, **10**, 407–409.

Netter, F. H. (1983) *Farbatlanten der medizin*, Thieme Verlag: Stuttgart, New York.

Sandritter, W. (Ed.) (1987) *Allgemeine Pathologie*, 2nd edition, Schattauer: Stuttgart, New York.

Thomas, C. (1987) *Makropathologie*, 7th edn, Schattauer: Stuttgart, New York.

Thomas, C. (1986) *Histopathologie*, 10th edn, Schattauer: Stuttgart, New York.

Thomas, C. (Ed.) (1988) *Bilddokumentation*. Deichert, L. and Thomas, C. (1988) 'Arteriitis temporalis Horton', *Med. Welt*, **39**, 1–3.

Thomas, C. (Ed.) (1987) *Bilddokumentation*. Rueschoff, J., Heide, M. and Thomas, C.: 'Angeborener Verhofseptumdefekt — paradoxe Embolie', *Med. Welt*, **38**, 1429–1432.

Thomas, C. (Ed.) (1987) *Bilddokumentation*. Gorenfloh, M., Rueschoff, J. and Thomas, C. 'Zur pathomorphologie der dilatativen (kongestiven) Kardiomyopathie', *Med. Welt*, **38**, 322–324.

Thomas, C. (Ed.) (1985) *Internationales Lehrbuch für Pharmaberater*. Kalbfleisch, H.: Das Herz-Kreislaufsystem. Part 1. Schattauer: Stuttgart, New York.

Thomas, C. (Ed.) (1985) *Internationales Lehrbuch für Pharmaberater*. Hombach, H., Das Herz-Kreislaufsystem. Part 2. Schattauer: Stuttgart, New York.

Thomas, C. (Ed.) (1982) *Infektionskolleg in Wort und Bild. Chirurgische Entzuendungen*. Roeher, H.-D., Thomas, C. and Dombrowski, H., Schattauer: Stuttgart, New York.

Thomas, C. (Ed.) (1982) *Infektionskolleg in Wort und Bild*. Korting, G. W., *Hautentzuendungen*, Schattauer: Stuttgart, New York.

Thomas, C. J. and Kracht, J. (Eds) (1984) 'Forum Pathologicum'. Nilles, M. Wehr and Koehler, F. 'Adriamycin-Kardiomyopathie', *Med. Welt*, **35**, 103–108.

1 Introduction

1.1 THE CARDIOVASCULAR SYSTEM

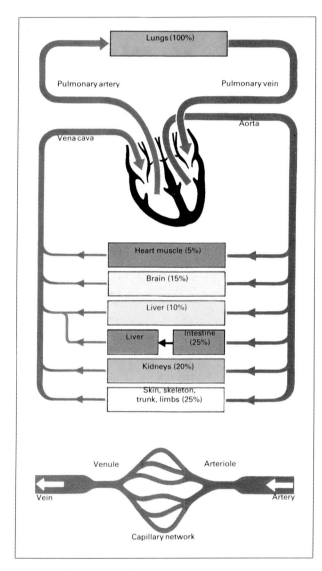

Fig. 1.1 Cardiovascular system.

The cardiovascular system (Fig. 1.1) consists of the heart together with the vessels of the general circulation (systemic circulation) and with the vessels of the lungs (pulmonary circulation). The components of the heart include the atrial and ventricular chambers, which are lined with endocardium, the heart valves, a muscular wall (myocardium) and an outer sac surrounding the heart (pericardium).

The large arteries act as conduction or distribution vessels to the microcirculation in the vascular beds. Here, there is an ordered arrangement of blood vessels with the small arterioles linking to the capillary networks before draining back to the heart through a system of venules which join the large veins. The structure of the cardiovascular system and the distribution of cardiac output to the various organs of the body under resting conditions is shown diagrammatically in Fig. 1.1.

The lymphatic system is also involved in the circulation of fluid. Lymphatic fluid is removed from the interstitium via the lymphatic capillaries, which drain into larger lymph vessels and their associated lymph nodes before finally entering collecting vessels which empty into the large veins of the upper body.

1.2 FUNCTION

The function of the cardiovascular system, or rather the blood circulating in it, is to exchange building and fuel material, metabolic products, heat and messenger substances among the various organs and tissues, and also between the body and the environment. This transport function is a prerequisite for the maintenance of homeostasis, which is essential for the normal function of cells, i.e. constancy of electrolyte concentrations, partial pressure of gases and temperature of the interstitial fluid.

1

2 Anatomy

2.1 TOPOGRAPHY

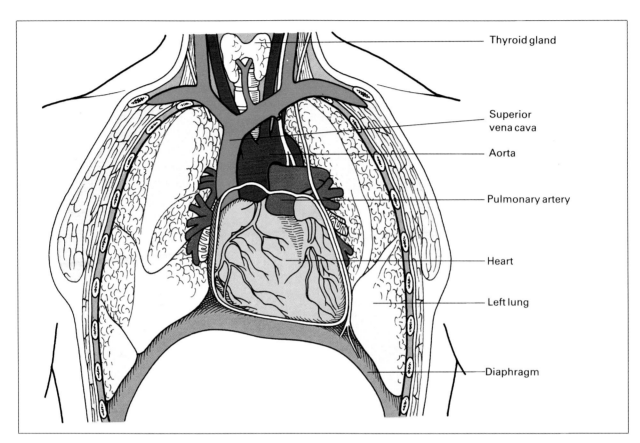

Thyroid gland

Superior vena cava

Aorta

Pulmonary artery

Heart

Left lung

Diaphragm

Fig. 2.1 Topography of the heart.

The heart is a roughly conical hollow muscle which, in adults, is composed of two separate halves, the right and left heart. The two halves are separated from one another by a dividing partition, the atrial and ventricular septum. Each half of the heart is further subdivided into an atrial and ventricular chamber and between each atrium and ventricle is a valvular opening that allows blood to flow only in the direction of the ventricle. There are also valves (semilunar valves) at the outlet from the heart where the great arteries begin (Fig. 2.1). These valves prevent the back-flow of blood from the arteries into the ventricles. The blood supply to the structures of the heart itself is maintained by coronary arteries and veins.

2.1.1 Site

The heart lies in the anterior part of the lower thorax, predominantly to the left of the mid-line. Most of the right and posterior wall lies on the central part of the diaphragm. Its main axis is tilted forwards and to the left, so that the apex is located anterior to the rest of the heart. The apex beat of the heart is usually located at the level of the left 5th intercostal space (5th ICS) in the mid-clavicular line. In many people, the apex beat can be seen and felt in this area. The great arteries run vertically upward in the mid-line. The great veins form a cross; the systemic veins run vertically and the pulmonary veins run horizontally. The anterior surface of the heart is largely overlapped by the lungs so that only a small section is not covered. In this area, the pericardium abuts directly on to the anterior chest wall.

2

2.1.2 Pericardium

The heart is contained within a fibro-serous sac, the pericardium. It has two layers which can be visualized by considering the heart as a ball which has been invaginated into a balloon of pericardium. The inner layer of the pericardium is in direct contact with the outer surface of the heart, extending as far as the origins of the great vessel and is then turned back as the outer layer or parietal pericardium. The two layers of the pericardium are lined with serous cells (mesothelial cells) which produce a small quantity of lubricating fluid, allowing the heart to move freely within the parietal pericardium. The most external layer of the pericardium forms a tough fibrous sheet which is attached to the sternum, the vertebral column and the diaphragm.

2.2 DISSECTION OF THE HEART

Dissection of the heart begins with a Y-shaped opening of the pericardium. Usually, about 10ml of a clear amber-coloured liquid is found in the pericardial sac. The inner surface of the pericardium is smooth, glistening and moist. The ventricles make up most of the anterior aspect of the heart. The anterior interventricular branch of the left coronary artery runs a straight course, enclosed in copious subepicardial fatty tissue in the anterior coronary sulcus. A circumscribed, whitish thickening is occasionally found on the anterior side of the right ventricle and is attributed to local mechanical irritation.

The heart can be opened in situ or after removal from the thorax by severing the aorta, pulmonary artery, pulmonary veins, and the inferior and superior venae cavae. Five incisions are made (Fig. 2.2):

1. Opening the right atrium: an incision is made with intestinal scissors from the inferior vena cava through the right atrium to the superior vena cava.
2. Opening the right ventricle: the second incision is made through the tricuspid valve to the apex of the right ventricle.
3. Opening the outflow tract of the right ventricle: a cut is made from the apex of the right ventricle through the pulmonary valve (between the cusps) and into the pulmonary artery.
4. Opening the left atrium: after cutting the pulmonary veins, an incision is made through the mitral valve to the apex of the left ventricle.
5. Opening the outflow tract of the left ventricle: this is achieved by a section from the apex of the

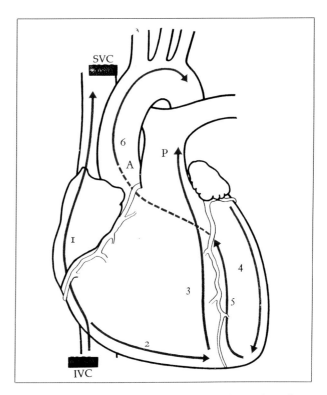

Fig. 2.2 Location of incisions (1–5) for dissection of the heart.
SVC: superior vena cava.
IVC: inferior vena cava.
A: aorta (6).
P: pulmonary trunk.

ventricle through the aortic valve (without disrupting the semilunar cusps) and into the aorta (6).

2.2.1 Coronary arteries

The left coronary artery (main stem, left anterior descending and left circumflex branches) is first sectioned from the ostium to the periphery. The right coronary artery is opened from the edge of the right ventricular incision to its ostium or to the apex of the ventricle.

2.2.2 Myocardial section

To examine the myocardium, incisions are made through the anterior and posterior wall of the left ventricle, parallel to the endocardium. The ventricular septum lies in the middle after the heart cavities have been opened. This forms two acute-angled triangles with the apices formed by the anterior walls of the right and left ventricles. The atrioventricular valves, with the atria and the out-

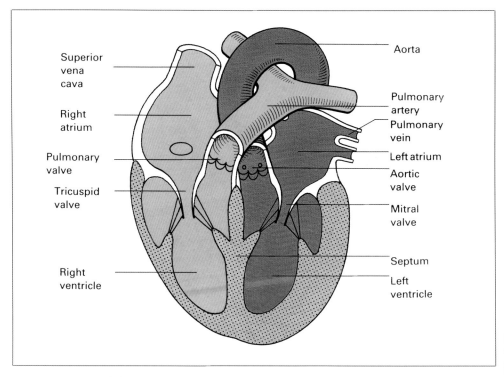

Fig. 2.3 Atria and ventricles of the heart.

Superior vena cava

Right atrium

Pulmonary valve

Tricuspid valve

Right ventricle

Aorta

Pulmonary artery

Pulmonary vein

Left atrium

Aortic valve

Mitral valve

Septum

Left ventricle

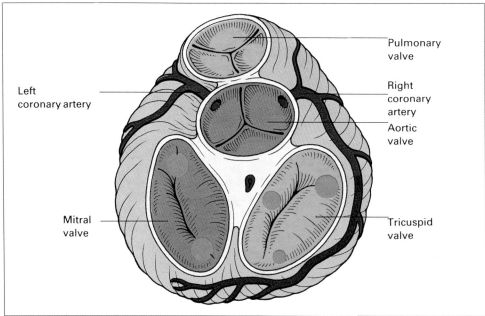

Fig. 2.4 Heart valves.

Left coronary artery

Pulmonary valve

Right coronary artery

Aortic valve

Mitral valve

Tricuspid valve

flow tracts of the ventricles and their associated semilunar valves, can be examined by displacing the apices.

2.2.3 Examination of the heart

Examination of the heart begins with examining its position within the thorax. The shape, size and weight of the organ, as well as the appearances of the pericardium and epicardium, are then assessed. After opening the heart, the following should be examined:

Appropriate course and communications of the great arteries and veins and coronary vessels.

Atria: width, endocardium, presence of thrombus, atrial appendage, foramen ovale.
Atrioventricular valves: circumference, cusps (deposits, scars, thickness), chordae tendineae (length, thickness).
Ventricles: wall (thickness, scars), chamber size, contents, trabecular musculature, endocardium.
Semilunar valves: circumference, state of the cusps (deposits, scars, outgrowths on the free margin, perforations).
Coronary arteries: pattern of supply (origin and course of the posterior descending branch), arterial lumen (width, presence of atheroma, thrombosis).
Myocardium: consistency, colour, presence of scars or deposits.

2.3 ANATOMY OF THE HEART

2.3.1 Dimensions

The size of the heart depends not only on its weight but also on the amount of blood which it contains. Generally, the size of the heart roughly corresponds to the size of the fist of the person concerned. The weight of the heart in a healthy adult is about 300–350g, which is 0.5% of the body weight. The end-diastolic internal volume of the ventricles is 270ml, and its greatest dimensions are 15 × 11 × 9cm. The dimensions of the heart under physiological conditions depend on body weight, age, sex and physical training. With intensive physical training, the weight of the heart may increase up to 500g ('athletic heart').

The heart is divided into two functionally separate units, the right and left heart. It can be further described as having an apex, and a base where the main blood vessels begin. The two atria are separated by a thin partition, the atrial septum, and the ventricles are divided by a thick muscular wall, the ventricular septum (Fig. 2.3). There is, therefore, no direct communication between the chambers of the left and right sides of the heart after birth. In the foetus, there is an opening in the atrial septum (foramen ovale) which allows blood to pass directly from the right atrium into the left atrium, bypassing the still unused pulmonary circulation.

The atria receive blood from the systemic and pulmonary veins. The superior and inferior venae cavae and the coronary veins, by way of the coronary sinus, open into the right atrium. The left atrium receives oxygenated blood returning from the lungs through four pulmonary veins. The ventricles have a thick muscular wall and represent the main driving force of the blood's circulation.

Within the ventricles, the flow of blood can be divided into a filling phase and an emptying phase. The great arteries arise from the outlets of the ventricles with the pulmonary artery on the right and the aorta on the left.

Dimensions and weights

Heart weight:
Men	300–350g
Women	250–300g
Abnormal weight	over 500g

Relative weight
(body weight) 0.5%

Child:
6 months	17–22g
12 months	30–40g
2 years	55–65g
5 years	85–95g
10 years	130–150g

Circumference of heart valves:
Mitral	9–11cm
Aortic	7–8cm

Thickness of ventricular wall:
Right ventricle	2–3mm
Left ventricle	12mm

(The thickness of the left ventricular wall is approximately 1/10th of the systolic pressure.)

Ratio between right and left ventricular wall:
Normal	2.3–3.3:1
Right ventricular hypertrophy	<2:1
Left ventricular hypertrophy	>3.3:1

Post-mortem ventricular volumes*:
Right ventricle	up to 25ml
Left ventricle	up to 10ml

*Depending on whether the ventricles are in systole or diastole and the presence of post-mortem clotting.

2.3.2 Heart valves

The atria and ventricles (Fig. 2.4) are separated from each other by rings of connective tissue (annuli fibrosi), with their associated valves. The left atrioventricular valve (mitral valve) has two cusps, whereas the right atrioventricular valve (tricuspid valve) has three. When the ventricles are relaxed in diastole, these valves open, allowing blood to flow

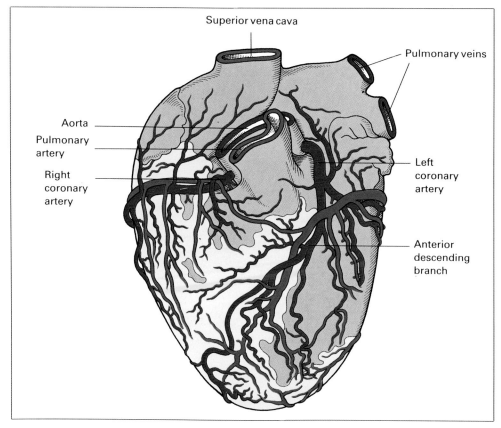

Fig. 2.5 Course of the coronary vessels. Anterior surface of the heart. (Coronary arteries red, coronary veins blue.)

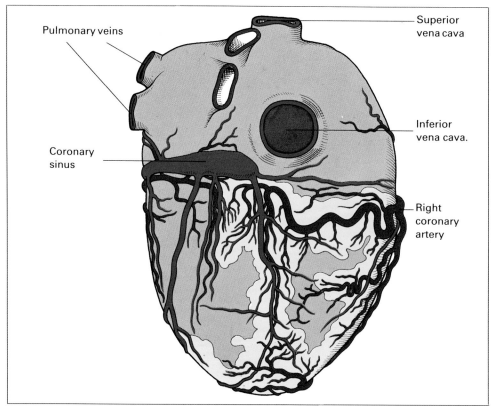

Fig. 2.6 Coronary vessels on the posterior surface of the heart. (Coronary arteries red, coronary veins blue.)

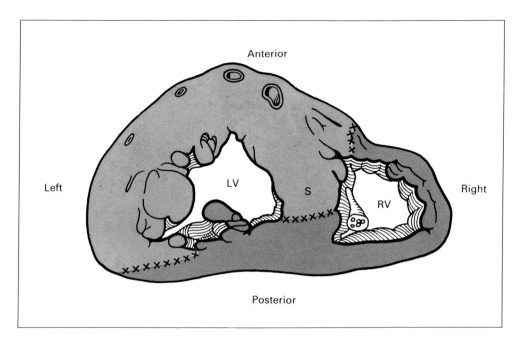

Fig. 2.7 Blood supply to the myocardium.
Blue: Left coronary artery.
Red: Right coronary artery.

LV: Left ventricle.
RV: Right ventricle.
S: Septum

from the atria into the ventricles. When the ventricles contract (systole) the mitral and tricuspid valves close, preventing regurgitation of blood back into the atria. Strong cords of fibrous tissue (chordae tendineae) are attached to the free margins of the valve cusps, preventing the valves prolapsing back into the atria under the force of ventricular contraction. In turn, the chordae tendineae are attached to the papillary muscles, which have the additional function of actively participating in the opening of the atrioventricular valves.

The semilunar valves are found at the origin of the great arteries, each consisting of three semilunar cusps. Behind each cusp, the arterial wall bulges outward, forming a pouch-like dilatation called the sinus of valsalva. During systole, when the ventricles contract, the pressure of blood forces the valve cusps open, passively pressing the cusps against the arterial walls and allowing the stream of blood to flow past. In diastole, when the ventricles relax, the column of blood begins moving back towards the heart and is caught in the sinus of Valsalva and passively presses the valve cusps shut.

2.4 CORONARY VESSELS

The continuous activity of the heart as a muscular pump requires a continuous supply of oxygen and nutrients. This is provided by the left and right coronary arteries which originate as the first branches of the aorta immediately above the aortic valve.

2.4.1 The left coronary artery

This divides into two main branches. The left anterior descending artery is a direct continuation from the left main coronary artery. It descends in the anterior interventricular sulcus to the apex of the left ventricle. It gives off diagonal branches which supply the anterior wall of the left ventricle and several septal branches which split off at right-angles to the main vessel (Fig. 2.5). The circumflex artery branches off the left main coronary artery at an obtuse angle and turns posteriorly as it runs around the left side of the heart in the atrioventricular sulcus. Its lateral branches supply the anterior and lateral walls of the left ventricle and the lateral parts of the posterior wall of the left ventricle.

2.4.2 The right coronary artery

This runs to the right in the atrioventricular sulcus, curving backwards around the edge of the right ventricle and crossing the posterior wall until it

7

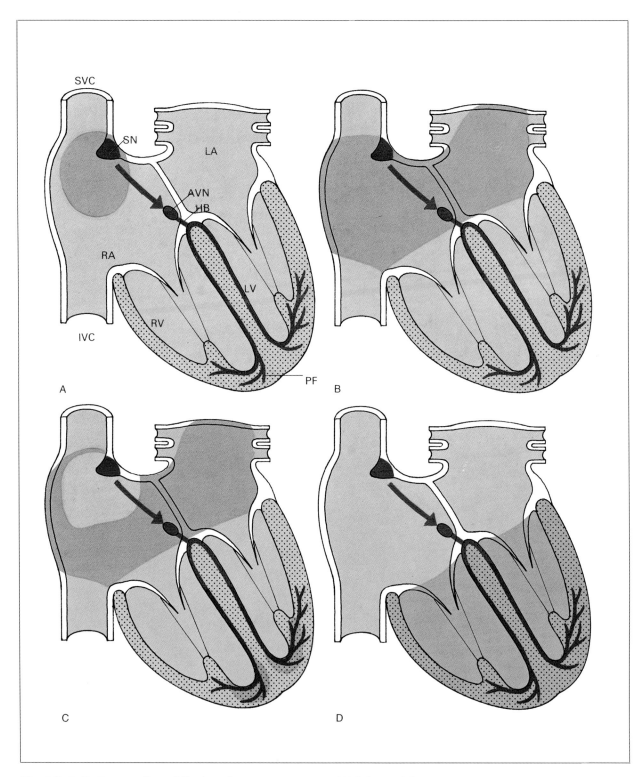

Fig. 2.8 A–D: Propagation of the impulse.
SVC: superior vena cava.
IVC: inferior vena cava.
RA: right atrium.
LA: left atrium.
RV: right ventricle.
LV: left ventricle.
SN: sino-atrial node.
AVN: atrioventricular node.
HB: Bundle of His with right and left branches.
PF: Purkinje fibres.

descends in the posterior interventricular sulcus. It supplies the entire right ventricle and the median portion of the posterior wall of the left ventricle. The right coronary artery and the left circumflex branch form a vascular ring encircling the heart. The left anterior descending artery and right posterior descending branches give off fine collateral vessels which form a broad vascular ring around the apex of the heart. Further collaterals are found over the ventricular septum but are only partially developed in the normal heart, so that the coronary arteries must be considered as functional terminal arteries. Coronary blood flow occurs predominantly during ventricular diastole as the arteries running within the myocardium are compressed during ventricular systole and blood flow ceases.

Venous blood is continuously fed back through the coronary veins which run parallel to the arterial branches (Fig. 2.6). They drain into the main collecting vessel, the coronary sinus, which opens into the right atrium.

2.4.3 Types of coronary supply (Fig. 2.7)

1. Balance type (70% of all hearts): the left coronary artery supplies the left heart with the exception of the posterior wall near the septum and the anterior two-thirds of the septum. The posterior descending artery arises from the right coronary artery.
2. Left dominant type (20%): the left heart and the entire septum are supplied by the left coronary artery. The posterior descending branch arises from the left coronary artery.
3. Right dominant type (10%): the anterior wall and the anterior two-thirds of the septum are supplied by the right coronary artery. The posterior descending branch runs to the left from the coronary sulcus.

2.5 THE CONDUCTION SYSTEM

In contrast to skeletal muscle which requires stimulation by signals originating in the central nervous system and conducted along motor nerves, the myocardium has the ability to create and propagate electrical signals itself. The efferent cardiac branches of the autonomic nervous system (sympathetic and parasympathetic) have only a modulating influence on impulse formation and conduction within the heart. Fibres of the vagus nerve innervate the atria, including the sinus node and atrioventricular node, but there is only a small input to the ventricles. The sympathetic fibres form a dense network in the atrial and ventricular musculature.

In the normal heart the impulses begin in the sino-atrial node, which is a specialized group of neuromyocardial cells located in the right atrial wall close to the confluence of the superior vena cava, right atrial appendage and the lateral wall of the right atrium. From there, the impulse spreads across the atrial musculature causing it to contract, and passes down to the atrioventricular node (AV node) in the floor of the right atrium (Fig. 2.8). The cardiac impulse then passes along the Bundle of His (a tract of specialized neuromuscular fibres), which crosses the fibrous ring at the atrioventricular junction and runs along the walls of the ventricular septum to the apex of the heart. The branches of the Bundle of His fan out as Purkinje fibres throughout the ventricular musculature causing them to contract.

At rest, the sino-atrial node generates 60–70 impulses per minute, establishing the normal heart rate. Normally the sino-atrial node initiates the cardiac impulse, but all parts of the conducting system are capable of forming stimuli. They act as a back-up should the sino-atrial node fail but have a lower frequency of impulse formation than the sino-atrial node.

2.6 HISTOLOGY OF THE HEART

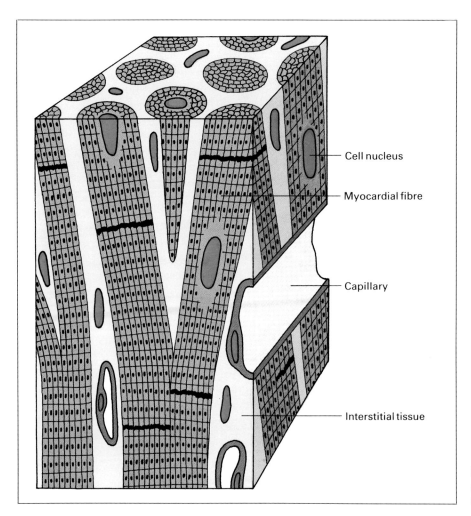

- Cell nucleus
- Myocardial fibre
- Capillary
- Interstitial tissue

Fig. 2.9 Histological structure of the myocardium.

The heart wall is composed of three layers: from inside to outside they are the endocardium, myocardium and epicardium.

The inner lining of the heart endocardium covers the inner surface of the ventricles and atria as well as the valves and chordae tendineae. It is composed of endothelial cells and a very thin connective tissue layer. Depending on the site, one can distinguish between parietal endocardium, which lines the heart chambers, and the valvular endocardium.

The greater part of the heart wall consists of muscle called myocardium (Fig. 2.9). It is thicker in the left ventricle than the right ventricle and only a thin layer in both atria. In dissection specimens, obliquely running, overlapping muscle fibres can be found winding in a spiral to the apex of the heart. The internal musculature forms columns, trabeculae and papillary muscles. The muscle cells are made up of striated fibres and are connected to each other in an interlinking network called the func-

tional syncytium. Anatomically speaking, it is not a true syncytium as the heart muscle cells are separated by cell membranes and are merely electrically coupled by numerous junctions. Each muscle cell is surrounded by capillaries which provide oxygen and energy supply for the uninterrupted work of the muscles. Specialized cells are capable of impulse formation and conduction and are known as the neuromyocardium.

The epicardium forms the outer surface of the heart. It is also the inner layer of the pericardium and is firmly attached to the myocardium. Its serous cells are covered with connective tissue, which serves as a lubricated sliding surface for the heart to move freely. Between the epicardium and the myocardium there is some subepicardial fatty tissue which evens out irregularities in the external heart contours, e.g. in the coronary sulci where the coronary vessels run between the two ventricles and between the atria and ventricles.

2.7   ULTRASTRUCTURE OF THE MYOCARDIAL CELL

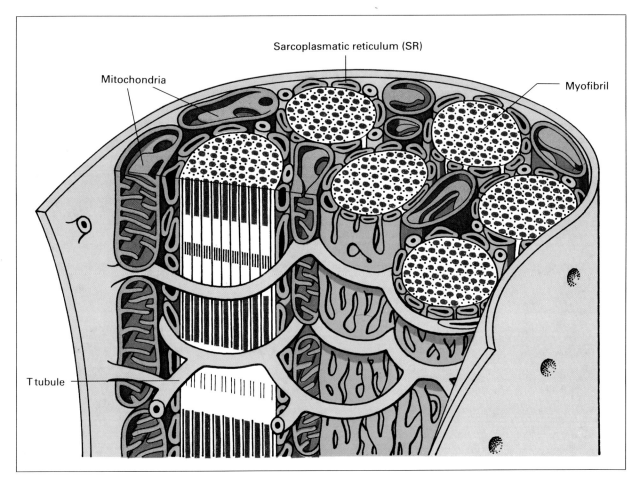

Fig. 2.10 Ultrastructure of the heart muscle cell. The myofibrils with their myofilaments (actin and myosin) represent the smallest contractile unit. They are surrounded by mitochondria (red) and the sarcoplasmatic reticulum (blue), which are the intracellular calcium stores.

The heart muscle fibres represent a functional syncytium where coordinated contraction occurs as a result of impulses spreading directly from cell to cell. Hundreds of cells are arranged longitudinally in series with multiple cells forming a fibre. The membrane of each muscle cell, the sarcolemma, has deep invaginations that form a branch system of tubules (T-tubules) running transversely between the myofibrils and mitochondria (Fig. 2.10). An electrical impulse (action potential) can be propagated through the T-tubules into the fibre interior. Another hollow cavity system running lengthways and in close contact (but without open connection) with the T-tubules is the endoplasmic of sarcoplasmic reticulum. This can store intracellular calcium ions which are released after stimulation and then actively re-uptaken. Numerous mitochondria lie between the myocardial fibrils and provide the

ATP necessary for contraction by oxidative metabolism.

The smallest contractile units are the sarcomeres which are linked end to end and side to side in large numbers. Intercallated discs are present at the junctions between sarcomeres, forming a specialized transversely running cell boundary. Within the sarcomeres are longitudinally running thick and thin protein filaments. The thick filaments are composed of myosin, and occupy the central part of the sarcomere, while the thin filaments of polymerized actin are at the ends. When a muscle fibre contracts, intermittent crossbridges are formed between actin and myosin filaments in the overlapping regions. This creates a ratchet effect, drawing the thin filaments in between the thick filaments and the whole sarcomere becomes shorter (sliding filament mechanism).

2.8 THE MAJOR SYSTEMIC ARTERIES

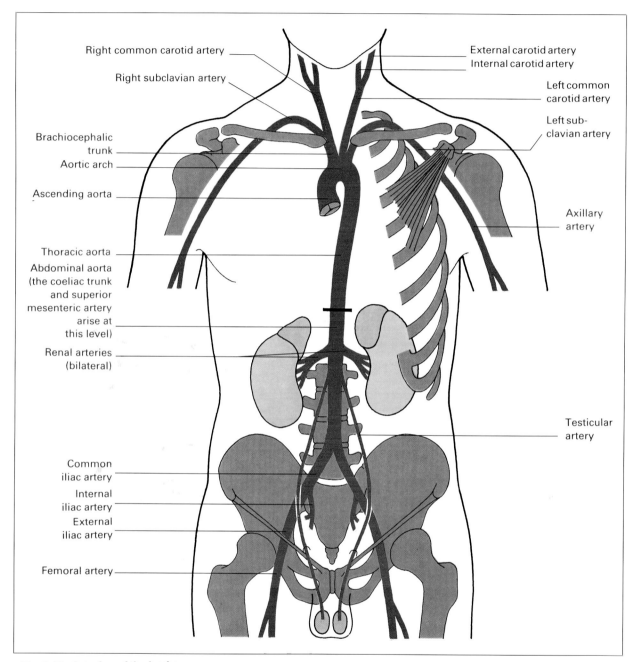

Fig. 2.11 Arteries of the body.

The arteries of the systemic circulation supply the organs, head and limbs and originate as branches of the aorta (Fig. 2.11). The aorta begins as an ascending trunk from the left ventricle (ascending aorta with the ostia of the coronary arteries), and then forms an arch which gives off the main arterial branches to the head and upper limbs (brachiocephalic trunk, left common carotid artery), before turning backwards and downwards as the descending aorta, with its thoracic and abdominal segments. It finally divides into the two common iliac arteries at the level of the pelvis.

The intercostal arteries are branches of the thoracic aorta, while the major branches of the abdominal aorta include the coeliac trunk (with the hepatic artery), the superior and inferior mesenteric arteries supplying the intestine, and the two renal arteries.

2.9 ARTERIES OF THE LIMBS (Fig. 2.12)

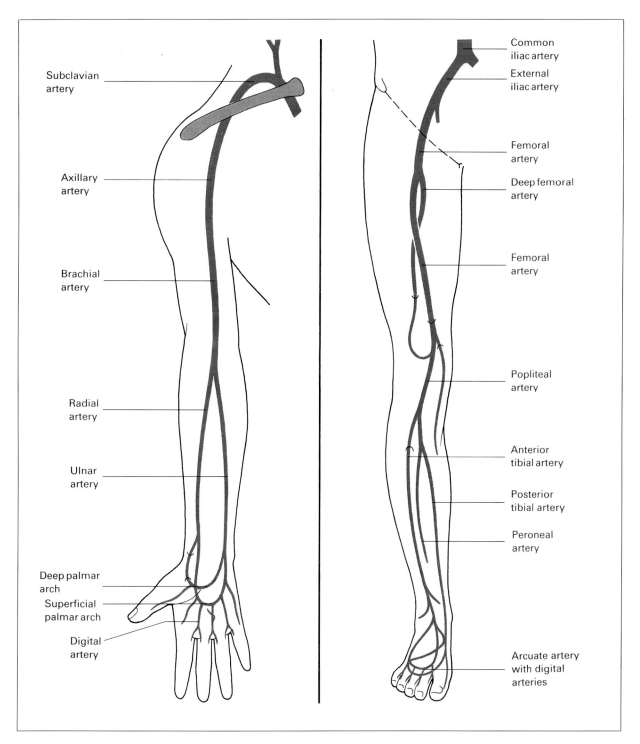

Fig. 2.12 Arteries of the upper and lower limbs.

13

2.10   THE MAJOR SYSTEMIC VEINS

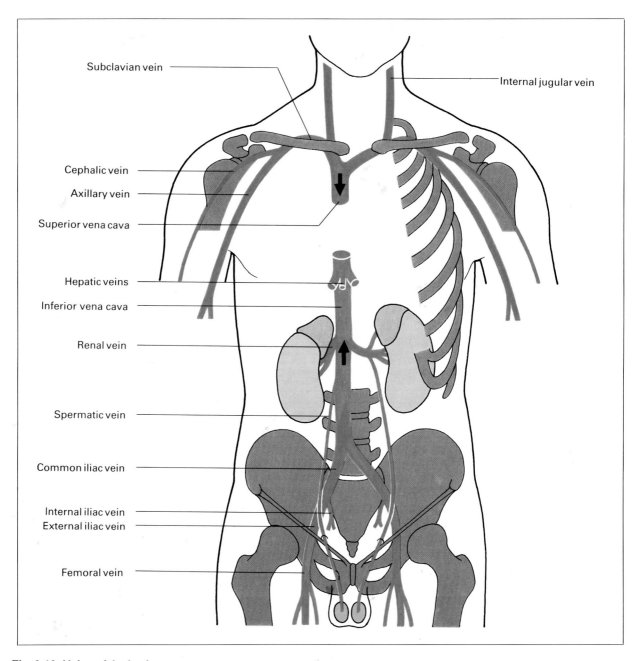

Subclavian vein

Internal jugular vein

Cephalic vein

Axillary vein

Superior vena cava

Hepatic veins

Inferior vena cava

Renal vein

Spermatic vein

Common iliac vein

Internal iliac vein
External iliac vein

Femoral vein

Fig. 2.13 Veins of the body.

The venous system of the systemic circulation forms a link between the capillary network and the right atrium (Fig. 2.13). Two large veins (superior and inferior venae cavae) return the desaturated blood from the upper and lower limbs, the head and the organs of the abdomen and chest. The venous drainage from the gastrointestinal tract, pancreas, spleen and liver is first collected by the portal circulation (via the portal vein), and passes through the liver before finally draining into the inferior vena cava.

2.11 VEINS OF THE LIMBS

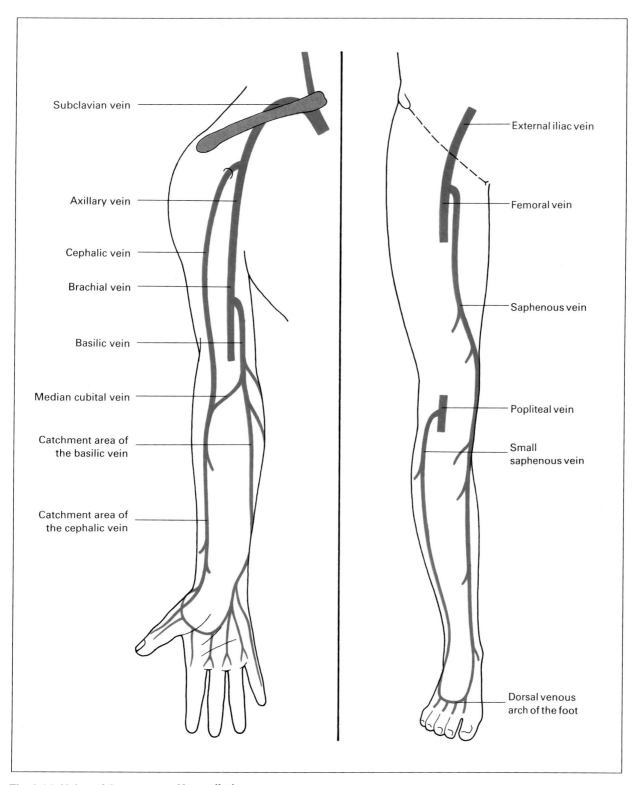

Subclavian vein

Axillary vein

Cephalic vein

Brachial vein

Basilic vein

Median cubital vein

Catchment area of
the basilic vein

Catchment area of
the cephalic vein

External iliac vein

Femoral vein

Saphenous vein

Popliteal vein

Small
saphenous vein

Dorsal venous
arch of the foot

Fig. 2.14 Veins of the upper and lower limbs.

The major veins of the limbs are shown in Fig. 2.14. They accompany the arteries and open into the superior vena cava or inferior vena cava.

2.12 HISTOLOGY OF THE BLOOD VESSELS

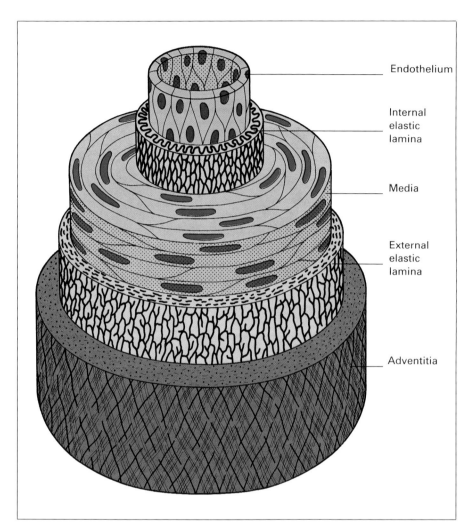

Endothelium

Internal
elastic
lamina

Media

External
elastic
lamina

Adventitia

**Fig. 2.15 Histological
structure of an artery.**

Blood vessels (arteries and veins) are the pipelines of the circulation, allowing the exchange of materials in the microcirculation where the capillaries are less than $30\mu m$ in diameter. Exchange between the blood and the interstitial fluid is facilitated by very thin walls in the microcirculatory vessels, the large surface area formed by the capillary network, and the associated slowing of blood flow as it is distributed through a large cross-sectional area of blood vessels. The interstitial fluid, which is present in variable amounts between the external capillary wall and the cells walls, is stabilized by mucopolysaccharides to form a jelly-like substance. Excessive fluid in the interstitium is drained off by the lymphatic system.

2.12.1 Arteries and veins

The structure of the vascular wall varies greatly depending on the site and function of the blood vessel, as well as the local blood pressure and the presence of normal or pathological conditions. Blood vessels are basically composed of three layers (Fig. 2.15).

1. The intima is the innermost layer and lines the vascular lumen. It is composed of flat endothelial cells arranged longitudinally along the length of the vessel and a thin connective tissue membrane enclosing occasional elastic and smooth muscle fibres.
2. The media is separated from the intima by an

16

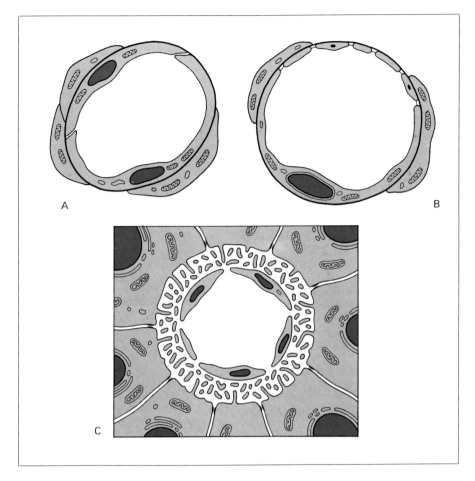

Fig. 2.16 Histological structure of the capillaries.
A) Closed type.
B) Normal type.
C) Sinusoid.

elastic layer (internal elastic lamina). The elastic fibres predominate in the large conduction vessels, such as the aorta and pulmonary arteries. Smooth muscle fibres predominate in the arterioles, providing the ability to regulate the blood flow into the capillary beds. Veins also have elastic muscle fibres in their walls but, compared with arteries, are thin walled and have a large lumen. The return of blood to the heart from the limbs is assisted by the presence of numerous venous valves in the moderately large limb veins, which prevents back-flow of blood to the periphery.

3. The adventitia is largely formed from collagen and elastic fibres which surround and support the vessels. It is separated from the media by a layer of elastic fibres (external elastic lamina), but they are not present in as great numbers as in the tunica elastica interna. The adventitia incorporates the vessel in the surrounding tissue and also contains the vessels (vasa vasorum) and nerves that supply the vascular wall itself.

2.12.2 Capillaries

The capillaries (3–8μm in diameter) are composed only of an endothelial layer supported by a basal membrane (Fig. 2.16). Depending on their function, three types are described:

1. Continuous capillaries: in these vessels, the lumen is separated from the surrounding tissue by overlapping endothelial cells and an intact basal membrane. Typically, they are found in the central nervous system.
2. Fenestrated capillaries have an intact basal membrane but pores between the endothelial cells which facilitate exchange between the capillary lumen and its surroundings. This is the most common type of capillary structure.
3. Sinusoids have walls with the greatest permeability. Large pores and the lack of a basal membrane allow free exchange with the surrounding tissues and are typically found in the liver.

17

2.13   ANASTOMOSES, COLLATERAL CIRCULATION AND TERMINAL BED

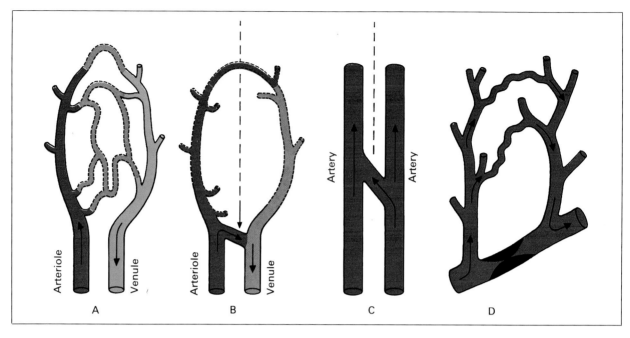

Fig. 2.17 Circulation.
A) Normal circulation.
B) Arteriovenous anastomosis.
C) Arterial anastomosis.
D) Collateral circulation in the case of arterial stenosis.

2.13.1 Anastomoses

Bypass vessels between some arteries and veins are designed to circumvent a capillary bed and are called arteriovenous anastomoses. There are also lateral communications between similar types of arteries running in parallel. These are also called anastomoses when they connect two arteries of different organ beds. Anastomoses occur regularly in the normal heart and increase in number in the presence of chronic coronary atheroma (Fig. 2.17).

2.13.2   Collaterals

A collateral is a connection between two segments of the same artery. Blood flows through the collateral channels to the distal vessel if the main artery becomes blocked and thus acts as a back-up supply route.

2.13.3   Terminal bed

The vascular system reaches its greatest surface area in the terminal bed. There are close to 2000 capillaries in 1mm^3 of myocardium. The diameter of a single capillary is 3–8μm. Blood flow in capillaries is intermittent and only a proportion of them open up at any one time. If increased blood flow is required, the percentage of perfused capillaries increases, and they can also increase in number by budding if intensive prolonged demands are made on the heart.

If there are no collaterals between arteries in a terminal bed, they are called terminal arteries. If some collaterals are present, but insufficient to take over complete supply to the local tissues should the main arterial lumen become occluded, the arteries are called functional terminal arteries. In the heart muscle, there are insufficient collateral vessels to take over the supply of blood to the myocardium in the event of sudden coronary occlusion. Thus, blockage of a major coronary artery results in extensive myocardial necrosis (tissue death). On the other hand, narrowing in the major coronary arteries is often a slowly progressive process, gradually leading to complete occlusion. This allows time for collateral vessels to develop in size and number and when the major vessel occludes, myocardial necrosis does not necessarily follow.

3 Physiology

3.1 FORMATION OF IMPULSES IN THE HEART

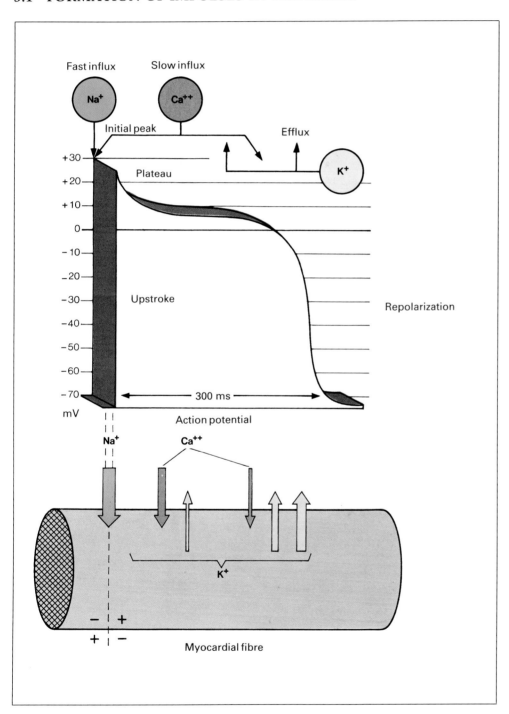

Fig. 3.1 Action potential of a myocardial fibre (top) with a diagram of the transmembrane ion fluxes during stimulation (bottom).

Under resting conditions, there is an electrical potential difference between the cell interior and the surroundings (resting membrane potential), and when the myocardial cell is stimulated, it can change the polarity of this transmembrane potential for brief periods (action potential).

3.1.1 Resting membrane potential

The myocardial cell creates the potential difference by forming concentration gradients of potassium, sodium and calcium ions between the intracellular and extracellular compartments. The intracellular potassium concentration is approximately 40 times higher than the extracellular concentration, whereas sodium concentration is about 20 times lower intracellularly, and that of calcium as much as 10 000 to 100 000 times lower. These gradients are created with the aid of active ion transport mechanisms (ion pumps) within the cell membrane.

Cardiac cells have a large transmembrane voltage under resting conditions of about −60 to −90 millivolts. If there were no voltage gradient across the membrane, the movement of potassium ions across the cell membrane would be determined solely by the concentration gradient. However, fixed negative charges within the cell (proteins and polypeptides), which are too large to diffuse out of the cell, attract potassium ions and impair their outward movement.

In the resting state, the myocardial cell membrane is most permeable to potassium. The flow of potassium ions out along its concentration gradient would make the charge within the cell interior more negative and create an electrical driving force for the influx of positively charged potassium ions. When the chemical and electrical forces balance out and the net flow of potassium is zero, the potassium equilibrium potential would be obtained at about 100 millivolts (interior negative). However, as the membrane is also permeable to some degree to sodium and calcium, the resting membrane potential moves to a less negative value of about −90 millivolts. Thus, the total flow of electrical charge through the membrane is zero, but small amounts of potassium still flow out and small amounts of sodium and calcium flow in. If the sodium ions were not extruded from the cell, the resting potential would decrease as sodium accumulated. Thus, the ion flow is continuously compensated for by cell membrane ion pumps. The energy for sodium pump is provided by ATP cleavage.

3.1.2 Action potential

The permeability of the myocardial cell membrane for the different ions depends on the membrane potential (Figs 3.1 and 3.2). Depolarization of the cell can be described in five phases. Either spontaneously, or in response to an external stimulus, sodium permeability across the cell membrane

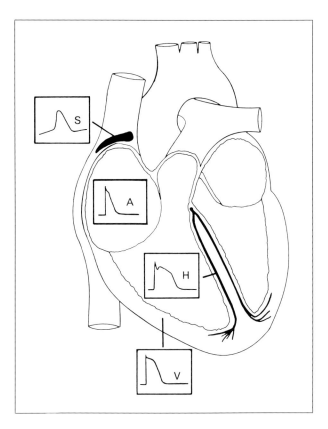

Fig. 3.2 Action potential curves in the cells of the sino-atrial node (S), atrial myocardium (A), Bundle of His (H) and ventricular myocardium (V).

increases greatly for a few milliseconds and raises the intracellular voltage above a critical threshold value. Once threshold level has been exceeded, sodium influx increases enormously and there is rapid depolarization of the cell to approximately +30 millivolts (rapid depolarization, phase 0). As in skeletal muscle or nerve cell membranes, the activated sodium system is turned off again within a few milliseconds and sodium influx suddenly ceases. This accounts for an early repolarization from the peak of the action potential to a notch at around +10 millivolts (phase 1). Depolarization also induces a considerable but, compared with the sodium system, slower increase in calcium permeability which counteracts the repolarization and creates a plateau or gently downward-sloping part of the action potential (phase 2). After inactivation of this slow calcium movement, there is increasing outward potassium flux leading to a negative charge inside the cell and the membrane potential returns to its resting value (repolarization, phase 4).

3.1.3 Regional differences

In different areas of the conducting system, the nature and time course of the complex changes in ion permeability which occur during the action potential, differ. In the sinus node, the fast sodium influx at the start of the action potential is largely missing and the upstroke is correspondingly much slower. The basis for slow potentials is an ionic channel which is selectively permeable to calcium ions which both opens and inactivates slowly. The duration of slow calcium influx is longest in the neuromyocardial cells of the Bundle of His and the Purkinje fibres. In the working myocardium of the ventricle, calcium influx is much longer than in the atrial myocardium and thus the action potential is correspondingly longer as well.

3.1.4 Refractory phase

When the heart muscle fibre is highly depolarized (action potential plateau phase 2), the sodium system which initiates the stimulus cannot be reactivated. The myocardial cell is therefore insensitive to further electrical depolarization during the plateau phase (absolute refractory period) and for a short period afterwards is sensitive only to a limited degree (relative refractory period). The duration of the plateau and thus of the refractory phase determines the maximum frequency of contraction that can be achieved by the heart muscle fibre. Atrial myocardium can beat at a higher frequency than that of the ventricle, but the particularly prolonged action potential and refractoriness in the neuromyocardial tissues of the ventricles protect against excessively high frequency stimuli originating in the atria.

3.1.5 Autonomous impulse formation

All regions of the neuromyocardial conducting tissue and, under certain circumstances, even the fibres of the working myocardium are able to initiate stimuli and contractions spontaneously. This automaticity takes place as a result of spontaneous depolarization of the muscle cell membrane. Starting from the end of repolarization, the membrane potential never rests at a stable value, but undergoes slow depolarization until after some time the threshold level is reached which triggers rapid influx of sodium and/or calcium and the action potential begins. The spontaneous depolarization occurs as a result of complex changes in the membrane permeability for various ions, which occurs differently in different regions. In the sinus node, an increase in the slow influx of positively charged calcium ions is of particular importance, whereas the spontaneous depolarization of Purkinje fibres is mainly due to a decrease in potassium permeability, causing a decrease in the efflux of positive charge. Through these various mechanisms, the threshold for depolarization is reached after a shorter or longer time. The sinus node has a much faster rate of spontaneous depolarization than the His–Purkinje system and, as the primary pacemaker, takes control of the cardiac rhythm. The electrical signals arising in the sinus node spread through the atria to the atrioventricular node and, from there, pass along the Bundle of His and the Purkinje fibres. The action potentials from the sinus node reach these regions before their own spontaneous depolarization reaches threshold levels. Only if the sinus node is diseased, or conduction fails, do other areas of the neuromyocardial conducting tissue take over control of heart rhythm. Heart rate will then fall from 60–80/min (sinus rhythm) to 40–60/min if the AV node takes over pacemaker function, or even to 20–40/min if impulse formation begins in the Purkinje fibres.

3.2 IMPULSE PROPAGATION

From the sinus node, the impulse spreads at a speed of about 1m/s through the right atrium and, slightly later, through the left atrium. Atrial stimulation is completed within 60–80msec. After reaching the atrioventricular node, the speed of impulse propagation slows dramatically to 10–20cm/s so that its passage through the upper AV node region takes 60–100msec. This accounts for most of the PR intervals on the surface electrocardiogram. The neuromyocardial tissue of the Bundle of His and the Purkinje fibres then conduct the impulse very rapidly (2–4m/s) crossing this segment in 20–30msec. Thus, most of the endocardial surface of the ventricular musculature is activated almost simultaneously. Propagation of the impulse through the ventricular myocardium takes place at the same speed as in the atrium.

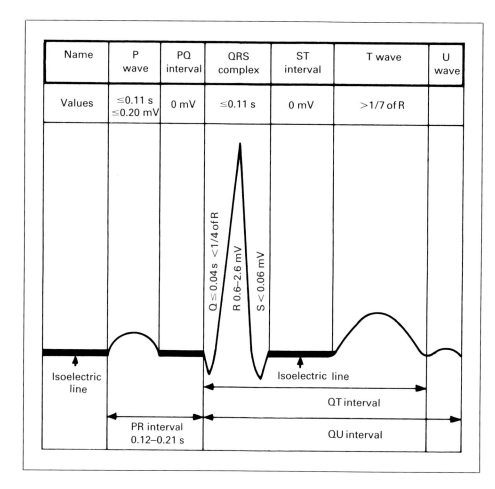

Name	P wave	PQ interval	QRS complex	ST interval	T wave	U wave
Values	≤0.11 s ≤0.20 mV	0 mV	≤0.11 s	0 mV	>1/7 of R	

Q ≤ 0.04 s < 1/4 of R

R 0.6–2.6 mV

S < 0.06 mV

Isoelectric line

Isoelectric line

QT interval

PR interval 0.12–0.21 s

QU interval

Fig. 3.3
Electrocardiogram
(standard limb leads).

3.2.1 Electrocardiogram (Fig. 3.3)

During the spread of an impulse from the sinus node, as well as during the subsequent repolarization phase, some regions of the myocardium are stimulated, others have yet to be stimulated and still others are no longer stimulated. As a result, the surface of stimulated myocardial fibres is negative (if the internal membrane potential is positive) in relation to the surface of unstimulated areas. Regional potential differences between the myocardial segments with good electrical conductivity (e.g. atrial myocardium and ventricular myocardium) act as electrical dipoles that can be transmitted through electrodes placed over the heart. The electrical fields spread over the entire body, which acts as a volume conductor, and the voltages can therefore be detected, although with reduced amplitude, on the body surface (electrocardiogram). The difference in the electrical potential between a fully stimulated atrium and an unstimulated ventricle (or vice versa) does not act as a potential difference that can be recorded on the surface electrocardiogram, since these myocardial regions are only connected through the relatively high resistance of the Bundle of His. Phases of this type therefore appear on the electrocardiogram, on the isoelectric line, in the same way as in a resting phase. The initial impulse formation within the sinus node cannot be detected on the surface ECG, but the propagation of the impulse through the atria results in the P wave. During the following PQ interval, the atria are fully stimulated and the impulse passes through the atrioventricular node and the Bundle of His and can be detected only by direct intracardiac electrocardiography. The depolarization of the ventricles is represented by the QRS complex and the very large change in electrical potentials at this time conceals the repolarization phase of the atria.

During the ST segment, the ventricular myocardium is fully stimulated and the atrial myocardium is fully repolarized. Finally, the T wave is due to repolarization of the ventricles.

The electrocardiogram provides clues to the pathway of stimulation in the atria and ventricles and may assist in the location of ischaemic or infarcted areas. It also shows characteristic changes when the transmembrane ion gradients are disturbed, e.g. in hyper- or hypokalaemia.

3.3 ELECTROMECHANICAL COUPLING

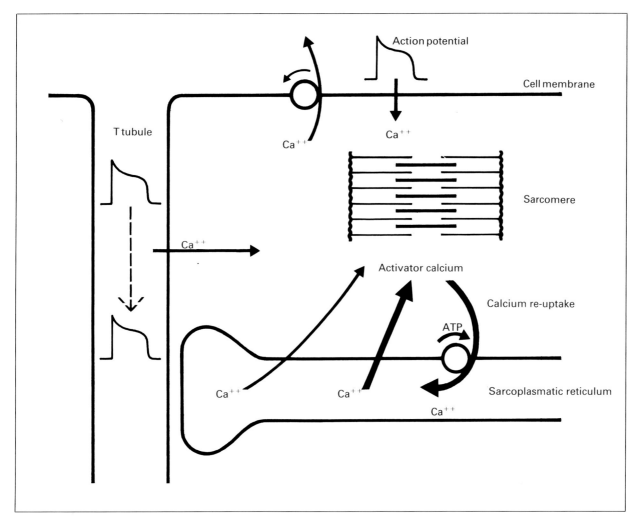

Fig. 3.4 Stimulation-contraction coupling in the myocardial fibre with interaction of actin and myosin via the calcium signal system.

The term electromechanical coupling summarizes the mechanisms whereby the stimulation of a cell membrane, resulting in the action potential, is converted into the activation of the sliding filament system of the contractile apparatus of the heart muscle fibres (Fig. 3.4). The interaction of actin and myosin filaments with the formation and shifting of crossbridges, leading to sarcomere shortening, is prevented in the unstimulated heart muscle fibre by a protein complex of tropomyosin and troponin located on the thin filaments. This inhibition is abolished when the intracellular concentration of free calcium ions increases, binding to receptors on troponin and changing their conformation. When the calcium concentration rises from normal values to 10^{-8}mol/l to over 10^{-6}mol/l, the contractile apparatus is switched on and later inactivated when the calcium concentration falls.

3.3.1 Step-by-step activation

The calcium level inside the cell is controlled by the sarcoplasmic reticulum. The membrane of this hollow system contains calcium transport proteins which, with the consumption of ATP, rapidly and effectively transport calcium ions inwards. When a propagated wave of excitation reaches the cell interior through the network of T-tubules running transversely through the fibres, the sarcoplasmic

23

reticulum is stimulated to release the calcium ions stored within it. Contraction is induced by the binding of free calcium ions to troponin and removes an inhibition on a configurational change in tropomysin, which, in turn, removes an inhibition to actin and myosin interaction. The result is to allow actin filaments to slide between myosin filaments, thus producing shortening. Relaxation is heralded by the transport of calcium ions back into the sarcoplasmic reticulum.

3.3.2 Contractile state

The amount of tension developed within the myocardial cell depends on the extent of calcium released from the sarcoplasmic reticulum. The calcium ion concentration in this storage system depends on the total calcium concentration of the myocardial fibre. During the action potential, both the sarcoplasmic reticulum membrane and the cell membrane with its invaginations, the T-tubules, becomes more permeable to calcium ions (slow calcium influx). As peak tension is being developed, the calcium pump on the sarcoplasmic reticulum is actually removing calcium from the cytoplasm and also into extracellular compartments by the calcium transport mechanism of the cell membrane. When the heart rate increases this is associated with greater release of calcium from the sarcoplasmic reticulum. When the heart rate increases, the period between action potentials (electrical diastole) is the phase which is particularly shortened, leading to a relative increase in the duration of the stimulation period of the action potential when calcium is released. Thus, increasing heart rate is associated with an increase in the contractile force of the heart, called frequency inotropism. This can be most clearly demonstrated in a heart that has stopped and is started up again. The first beats are weak as the intracellular calcium concentration is low during the previous relaxation phase due to outward transport of calcium. With each successive stimulation, more and more calcium ions are brought into the cell, so that the amplitude of contraction increases from beat to beat (staircase phenomenon). A similar phenomenon occurs when the calcium influx is increased by a premature additional stimulus (extrasystole). As a result of the increased intracellular calcium concentration with a premature stimulus, the next regular beat is stronger. This post-extrasystolic potentiation then fades away as the original flow

equilibrium is restored.

The degree of tension developed during cardiac contraction is dependent not only on external concentration of calcium but also on the length of the sarcomere. If the sarcomere becomes shorter, e.g. as a result of lowering end-diastolic volume, the amount of calcium available for release from the sarcoplasmic reticulum is reduced. Conversely, when the end-diastolic volume of the left ventricle increases, the force of contraction will also increase (Starling's law).

3.4 ENERGY METABOLISM OF THE HEART

The immediate source of energy for myocardial fibre contraction and for the ion transport mechanism that maintains the concentration gradients between the intra- and extracellular compartments or between the cytosomal and sarcoplasmic reticulum is the energy-rich phosphate ATP. Most of the necessary ATP is produced by the heart through oxidative phosphorylation in its mitochondria. The oxygen consumption of the myocardium is higher than all other organs in the body at approximately 9ml/min/100g. As substrates for ATP production, it extracts free fatty acids as well as glucose, lactate, pyruvate, ketone bodies and amino acids from the blood. Under resting conditions, glucose consumption accounts for one-third of the oxidative metabolism, but much less during exercise. Due to its ability to metabolize lactate, the heart makes a considerable contribution to the elimination of lactic acid produced by skeletal muscles during continuous aerobic exercise.

3.4.1 Anaerobic metabolism

Unlike skeletal muscle, energy production by anaerobic glycolysis is negligible in the heart muscle. In the presence of anoxia, e.g. after acute coronary occlusion, the heart muscle is unable to continue its activity for long. It can certainly beat for 6–10min after its oxygen supply has been cut off but is no longer able to maintain the blood pressure. If coronary perfusion has to be interrupted for prolonged periods, e.g. during coronary bypass surgery, cardiac metabolism must be reduced to a minimum level by inhibiting the automatic impulse formation (using a cardioplegic solution) and by cooling in order to prevent injury.

3.4.2 Oxygen requirement

The oxygen consumption of the myocardium is determined not only by its pumping action (pressure volume work) but also by the efficiency with which the oxidatively produced chemical energy is converted into mechanical work. This efficiency, which is normally about 10%, depends greatly on the conditions under which the heart is working. For equal pressure volume work, the efficiency is poorer and oxygen demand is greater if the blood pressure to be maintained is higher and the heart rate faster. For an incremental rise in contractile force, the oxygen requirements increase disproportionately. Increased workloads induced by an increase in arterial pressure result in greater oxygen demands than similar workloads induced by an increase in volume. Combined loads that result in increased pressure and output and in increased contractility, as during exercise, cause the greatest increments in myocardial oxygen requirements.

3.5 CORONARY PERFUSION

Although the heart muscle represents only about 0.5% of total body weight, it consumes 10–20% of the total oxygen taken in by the body. Myocardial blood flow is approximately 80ml/100g/min at rest, i.e. at the upper end of the range for working skeletal muscles. Coronary blood flow represents 4–5% of total cardiac output and even under resting conditions, oxygen extraction from coronary blood flow is almost maximal, so that the heart can only increase its oxygen supply during exercise by increasing coronary blood flow.

During exercise, coronary blood flow can increase by a factor of 4–5 times (coronary reserve). This increase in perfusion is brought about by a local chemically induced dilatation of the vessels, for which adenosine is considered to be responsible. Stimulation of the sympathetic supply to the coronary vessels causes vasoconstriction of the large arteries (alpha-receptor effect of noradrenaline), so that over-activity of the sympathetic system can produce neurally induced ischaemia (Prinzmetal's angina). However, the contribution of the large conductive vessels to the total vascular resistance is so small that constriction of the coronary lumen only becomes functionally significant when the diameter has been reduced by half.

Adequate perfusion of the ventricular myocardium is only possible during diastole, as arterial inflow ceases during ventricular contraction. In contrast, during systole, venous blood is squeezed out of the vascular bed. Arterial supply to the heart muscle deteriorates with increasing heart rate as a result of relative shortening of diastole, allowing less time for arterial inflow. This effect is particularly marked in the endocardial ventricular wall, which is directly exposed to the high internal ventricular pressure.

3.6 MECHANICAL ACTIVITY OF THE HEART

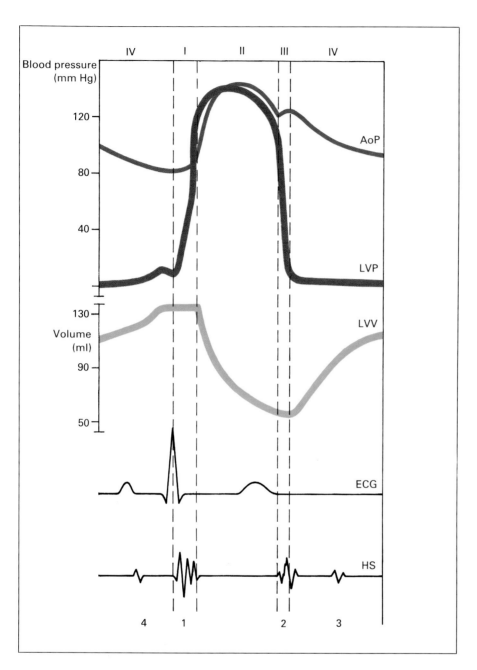

Fig. 3.5 Time curve of pressure in the ascending aorta (AoP) and in the left ventricle (LVP), and left ventricular volume (LVV) relative to the ECG and heart sounds (HS). The filling phase (IV), isometric contraction phase (I), ejection phase (II) and isometric relaxation phase (III) are noted at the top margin. The arabic numerals at the bottom designate the heart sounds.

The cardiac cycle includes a contraction phase or systole, and a relaxation phase or diastole. The term electrical systole, i.e. the period of membrane excitation, has a slightly different connotation from that of mechanical systole as the electrical events precede mechanical activity. Furthermore, atrial and ventricular systole do not coincide and, when used by itself, the word 'systole' usually refers to ventricular systole and especially that of the left ventricle. The QT interval on the surface ECG can be used as a guide to the duration of ventricular electrical systole.

3.6.1 Left ventricular systole (Fig. 3.5)

At the onset of mechanical systole, there is a rise in pressure in the left ventricle, which at this time contains about 130ml of blood. When the ventricular pressure rises above the pressure in the left atrium, the atrioventricular (mitral) valve closes producing the first heart sound. There then follows an isovolumetric contraction phase during which the ventricle exerts pressure on its contents until the internal ventricular pressure becomes higher than the pressure in the ascending aorta. At that point, the aortic valve opens and the systolic ejection phase begins. As the ventricle contracts, there is a further rise in intraventricular pressure, and blood is ejected at a peak of 1–2 m/sec. At about the middle of the ejection phase, there is a decrease in myocardial contractile force and the pressure inside the left ventricle begins to fall. Although intraventricular pressure drops below the aortic pressure during the second half of the ejection phase, the outflow of blood continues, maintained by its own kinetic energy. Then the direction of flow reverses and the aortic valve closes, preventing blood returning to the ventricle. The noise produced as the column of blood forces the aortic valve closed can be heard with the stethoscope as the second heart sound. In all, about half the volume of blood initially contained in the ventricle is ejected with each cardiac cycle (ejection fraction). The ejection fraction can increase during periods of increased myocardial contractility.

3.6.2 Right ventricular systole

The electrical impulse travelling along the conducting system reaches the right ventricular myocardium slightly later than the left ventricle, so that the start of the isovolumetric contraction phase of the right ventricle is also slightly delayed. None the less, the pulmonary valve opens earlier than the aortic valve as the diastolic pressure in the pulmonary artery is only about 10mmHg. Thus, contraction of the right ventricle causes opening of the pulmonary valve at considerably lower pressure than that necessary for the left ventricle to open the aortic valve (approximately 80mmHg). Consequently, the right ventricular ejection phase begins before left

ventricular ejection, but is of longer duration as the kinetic energy of the ejected blood maintains outflow against the lower resistance of the pulmonary vascular bed for a longer time before the direction of flow reverses. Thus, the pulmonary valve closes later than the aortic valve causing duplication or splitting of the second heart sound.

3.6.3 Ventricular diastole

Mechanical ventricular diastole starts with the isovolumetric relaxation phase after the aortic and pulmonary valves have closed but before the atrioventricular valves open. When the pressure inside the ventricles falls to about 5mmHg, the atrioventricular valves open and the ventricular filling phase begins. At a normal resting heart rate, ventricular filling occupies more than half the entire cardiac cycle, but with increasing heart rate, there is a relative shortening of diastole and ventricular filling time.

At rest, atrial contraction contributes little to overall ventricular filling (10–15%). As the ventricular filling phase shortens with increasing heart rate, the contribution of atrial systole to ventricular filling also increases. In patients with heart failure, blood driven from the atrium into the ventricle can be heard as a late diastolic fourth heart sound as the blood strikes the ventricular wall.

The stroke volume of the heart is determined both by the ejection fraction and the diastolic filling of the ventricles. If the heart rate is increased, the shortened filling time may initially be compensated by more rapid filling, which is assisted by the pressure suction pump action of the heart. During systole, the atrioventricular valve plane descends, facilitating venous return to the atria. When the ventricles relax, the valve plane springs back and may actually induce negative pressure in the ventricular cavity. This improves diastolic filling by the ventricles, so that almost complete emptying of the atria can occur. By this mechanism, heart rate can more than double without a significant decrease in stroke volume. Healthy persons aged between 20 and 30 years can increase their cardiac output from 5 l/min at rest to about 20 l/min during exercise, and top-class athletes can even reach an output of 30–40 l/min.

3.7   CONTROL OF CARDIAC OUTPUT

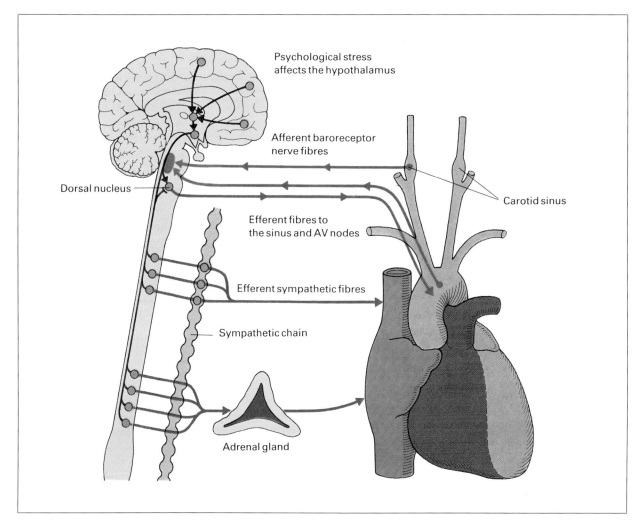

Fig. 3.6 Nerve pathways for control of the heart by the circulatory centre in the brain stem.

3.7.1   Autoregulation of the heart

Even without external controls, the heart is able to respond to changes in loading conditions resulting from increased venous return and associated diastolic filling (increased preload) or when there is increased resistance in the peripheral arterial vascular beds (increased afterload). When diastolic ventricular filling is increased, the resultant increase in left ventricular wall stress and stretching of the myocardial fibres is accompanied by a corresponding increase in the force of contraction. Stroke volume and cardiac output will therefore rise to adapt to the increased venous return. In physiological terms, this autoregulatory function is a trans-ient phenomenon and its main relevance is probably to balance the volumes emerging from the right and left ventricles. Since afterload influences the rate and extent of ventricular ejection, it will also influence the ventricular end-diastolic volume and subsequently the diastolic volume of the next cardiac cycle. Thus, in response to increased afterload, ventricular contractility will be enhanced.

3.7.2   Autonomic nervous control of the heart

The generation of impulses by the sinus node, together with the propagation of impulses along the conduction system and the rate and force of

28

contraction of the myocardium are influenced by the efferent cardiac nerves. The transmitter substance of the sympathetic nervous system is noradrenaline and that of the parasympathetic system (vagus nerve) is acetylcholine. These transmitter substances are released from the postganglionic nerve endings and bind to receptors in the myocardial cell membrane.

Sympathetic system

Noradrenaline binds to beta receptors on the cell membrane and induces a confirmation change in these receptors which, through several intermediate steps, leads to activation of the enzyme adenylcyclase on the internal side of the membrane. In turn, adenylcyclase catalyses conversion of adenosine triphosphate (ATP) to adenosine 3,5-monophosphate (cyclic AMP). This secondary messenger acts on the cell membrane so that its calcium channels allow more calcium ions through when depolarized. This results in an increased 'slow' calcium influx during the action potential. Increased intracellular calcium causes greater release of calcium ions from the sarcoplasmic reticulum when stimulated, resulting in increased myocardial contractility (positive inotropic effect). In the sinus node, enhanced slow calcium flow leads to faster spontaneous depolarization and, thus, an increase in heart rate (positive inotropic effect). The action of noradrenaline also leads to faster impulse propagation within the conducting system. At the same time, the ability of the cell membrane to conduct potassium during depolarization is increased by noradrenaline, so that repolarization starts more quickly despite the increased calcium influx, and the action potential duration is shortened, or at least remains the same. Relaxation of the heart muscle fibres after the stimulus has passed is also accelerated by sympathetic stimulation.

Parasympathetic system

Vagal fibres predominantly influence the atria and the specialized conducting tissue of the sinus node and the atrioventricular node, with only few vagal fibres reaching the ventricular myocardium. Acetylcholine released by the parasympathetic system primarily increases potassium flux across the myocardial cell membrane. Spontaneous depolarization is inhibited and repolarization starts earlier. Consequently, automatic impulse formation is slowed down (negative chronotropic effect), the conduction of impulses is delayed (negative dromotropic effect) and the excitability of the myocardium is generally depressed (negative bathmotropic effect). The decrease in contractility associated with the shortening of the action potential (negative inotropic effect) primarily affects the atrial myocardium and has only minimal influence on the ventricles. At rest, the influence of the parasympathetic system on the heart predominates over that of the sympathetic system. If the effects of all efferent cardiac nerves are interrupted, e.g. by drugs or after cardiac transplant surgery, resting heart rate is increased to approximately 100/min.

The action of the parasympathetic system on heart rate is more rapid (latent period 1–3s) than that of the sympathetic system (latent period 10–15s).

3.8 HIGHER NEURAL CONTROL (Fig. 3.6)

The control of cardiac function by the efferent nerves of the autonomic nervous system is controlled by a group of nerve cells in the brain stem, the circulatory centre. It receives information from superior brain segments (limbic system, hypothalamus), from pressure receptors in the vascular beds (carotid sinus, aortic arch, cardiac atria), from chemoreceptors in the blood stream (the carotid and aortic bodies which are sensitive to oxygen and carbon dioxide tensions) and from metabolic receptors which monitor skeletal muscle metabolism by recording changes in the interstitium, as well as impulses from the neighbouring respiratory centre. This information is evaluated in the circulatory centre and converted into control commands in the parasympathetic and sympathetic nerve cells. Rapid changes in heart rate are induced by the vagus nerve, whereas slower adjustments in heart rate and changes in contractility are caused by the sympathetic cardiac nerves and by the secretion of noradrenaline and adrenaline from the adrenal medulla.

3.9   SYSTEMIC CIRCULATION

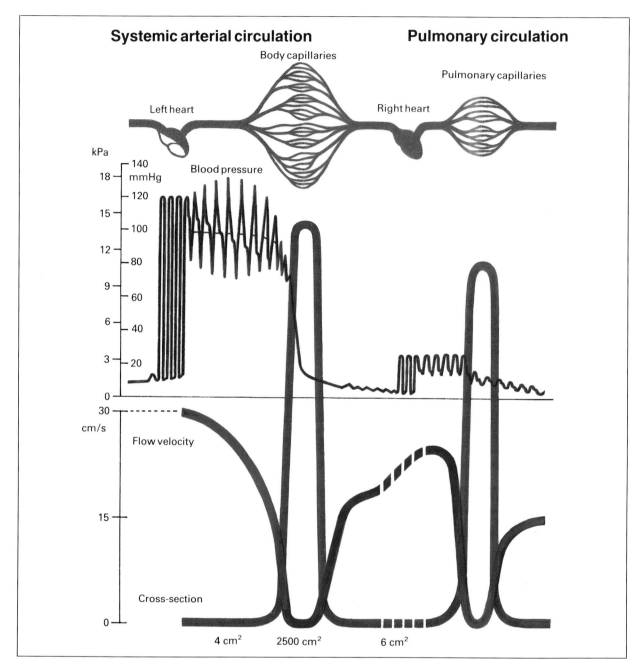

Fig. 3.7 Pressure, flow rate and total cross-section in the blood circulation.

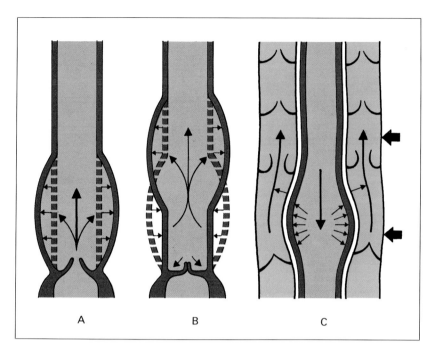

Fig. 3.8 A, B) Flow regulator function of the aorta. C) Venous return flow due to external pressure (pulsation of the accompanying artery or contraction of skeletal muscles).

3.9.1 Arterial segment

The left ventricle ejects its stroke volume into the aorta creating the pulse wave in the high-pressure part of the circulation. With a volume distensibility of about 1ml/mmHg, this first part of the arterial tree, with its elastic walls, acts as a flow regulator and stores about half the systolic stroke volume. The other half flows directly through the peripheral vascular resistance beds, mainly formed by the small arteries and arterioles, to reach the vessels of the microcirculation. As the blood passes through the large elastic arteries, the decrease in mean pressure is so slight, that it can be ignored in blood pressure measurement. Consequently, the blood pressure recorded by auscultation over the brachial artery can be considered equivalent to the systemic blood pressure. As the arterial pressure pulse wave passes to the periphery, there are significant changes in its form. At the end of ventricular systole, when the aortic valve closes, there is a brief recoil of blood causing an upward deflection in the arterial wave form. On its passage to the periphery the high-frequency portion of the pressure pulse is damped by wall friction, and a sign of this is the disappearance of the dicrotic notch. In the larger arteries, which are less elastic than the aorta, the pressure pulse is initially intensified so that peak systolic pressure in the femoral or radial artery is greater than the aorta, whereas the mean pressure is lower. The veins close to large arteries are locally compressed by the arterial pulse and, because of the presence of venous valves, venous compression facilitates peripheral return to the heart.

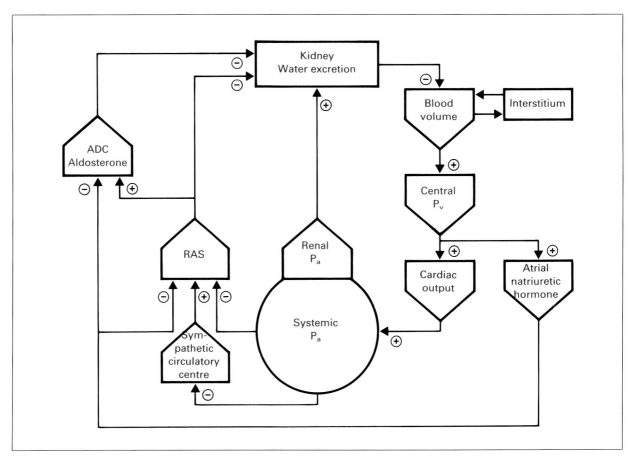

Fig. 3.9 Block diagram of the **regulation of systemic blood pressure** via effects of blood volume changes on venous return and thus on cardiac output. RAS: renin-angiotensin system. ADC: adrenal cortex.

3.9.2 Blood pressure regulation

The mean blood pressure in the systemic circulation is determined by the cardiac output and the peripheral vascular resistance. Peak systolic pressure is additionally influenced by stroke volume and the arterial distensibility. Arterial blood pressure is mainly regulated by the circulatory centre in the brain stem. This can both increase cardiac output and alter peripheral vascular resistance by activation of the sympathetic system to the local release of noradrenaline or the stimulation of adrenaline and noradrenaline secretion from the adrenal medulla. The parasympathetic system participates mainly in the control of heart rate since the parasympathetic innervation is of major functional significance in only a few vascular beds (sexual organs, lungs). To maintain arterial blood pressure at a fixed reference level determined by the higher influences from the brain, the circulatory centre utilizes information from the carotid sinus and the pressure receptors located in the aortic arch. A decrease in blood pressure within these vascular segments leads to counter-regulation starting within a few seconds (pressure receptor reflex).

The circulating blood volume has an important influence on blood pressure since the filling of the vascular beds determines the venous return and subsequently the cardiac output. Whereas the oxygen transport function of the blood depends on the eryythrocyte count, changes in plasma volume as a result of renal salt and water excretion are of overriding importance to blood pressure regulation. A complex series of interactions takes place between blood pressure and plasma volume regulation. When circulating volume is abnormally low and blood pressure falls, the renin–angiotensin–aldosterone system is activated, causing vasoconstriction and the retention of salt and water. When circulating volume is excessive, and arterial pressure is high, the atrial muscle cells respond to stretch by releasing atrial natriuretic peptide (ANP) which causes renal sodium excretion. Raised arterial pressure can also have a direct effect on kidney

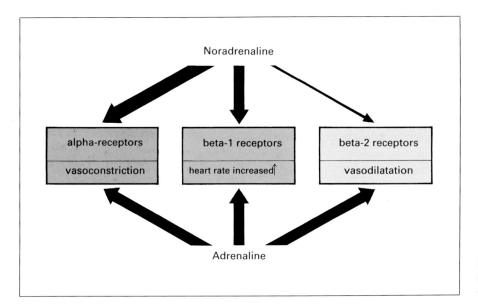

Fig. 3.10 Action of adrenaline/noradrenaline on receptors.

function through pressure diuresis. There are further links between control of blood pressure and control of blood volume through activation of the sympathetic nervous system which stimulates renal renin release in response to a fall in blood pressure.

3.9.3 Microcirculation

The exchange of heat, metabolic products and oxygen between the blood and the tissues takes place in the arterioles, capillaries and venules. Adjustment of blood perfusion to local requirements is achieved by local chemically controlled autoregulation of the arterioles. When arterial blood pressure changes, but the metabolic situation remains constant, a predominantly myogenic autoregulation system keeps blood perfusion constant, irrespective of pressure in many vascular beds (especially the kidneys, brain and skeletal muscles). The sympathetic nervous system plays an important role in altering regional blood flow in response to exercise. Vasoconstriction is mediated by alpha receptors and vasodilatation by the beta receptors. When the oxygen requirement of skeletal muscle increases during exercise, or when the circulating volume is reduced as a result of hypovolaemia or the erect posture, blood flow to the splanchnic bed and inactive muscles is reduced. The supply to vital organs, such as the heart and brain, is preferentially maintained, especially in conditions causing volume depletion. Vascular

innervation is also responsible for the adaptation of cutaneous blood flow to the skin to the requirements of thermoregulation (vasoconstriction in the cold, vasodilatation under warm conditions).

As the intraluminal pressure in the vessels is considerably greater than the interstitial pressure, even in the microcirculation, a hydrostatic driving force exists causing outward filtration of plasma. The colloidal osmotic pressure created by higher plasma protein concentration intravascularly, as compared with the interstitium, operates in the opposite direction. The excess fluid and protein filtered out into the interstitium are normally taken up by lymphatic capillaries and returned to blood in the lymphatic system. Excessive accumulation of fluid in the interstitium (oedema formation) can occur if the lymphatic pathways are obstructed, or if the transudation of plasma fluid from the blood vessel is in excess of the return, which can occur when the hydrostatic pressure is too great, e.g. in the feet during prolonged standing. It can also occur if the vascular wall permeability is too high or if the plasma protein concentration is too low.

Blood supply can be jeopardized if numerous vessels of the microcirculation become occluded. This typically occurs in disseminated intravascular coagulation (DIC), a phenomenon observed in some states of shock (particularly endotoxin shock), and is due to increased activation of the blood coagulation system by messenger substances of the defence system (including tumour necrosis factor and interleukin 1).

3.9.4 The capacitance vessels

The low-pressure part of the circulation, which includes the veins, venules and capillaries of the systemic circulation, the right heart, the pulmonary circulation, the left atrium and the left ventricle in diastole, contains about 85% of the total blood volume. Over three-quarters of this volume is found in the small veins and venules under physiological conditions. This low-pressure system has a volume distensibility (compliance) of about 200ml/mmHg. The blood pressure falls from 15–18mmHg in the small venules to about 5mmHg in the right atrium. The pressure in the right atrium and the largely similar pressure in the valveless superior inferior vena cava is called the central venous pressure (CVP). The CVP is the most important indicator of the blood volume in the capacitance vascular beds, which in turn is indirectly linked with systemic blood pressure. In hypovolaemia, the central venous pressure is low, and high in hypervolaemia and right heart failure.

Blood flow in the venules and veins is considerably slower and much more variable than that in the arteries. Veins are therefore susceptible to stasis if the minimal pressure gradient required to overcome the viscosity of the blood is not achieved. If flow stops, there is risk of clot formation (thrombosis).

Changing from the supine to the standing position exerts particular stress on the capacitance vessels. The hydrostatic pressure in the vessels of the foot and calf can increase to over 100mmHg on standing, even in the veins. Distension of the capacitance vascular beds in the dependent parts of the body and the outward filtration of plasma fluid can lead to accumulation of about 0.5l in the legs. To compensate for this loss of volume, vasoconstriction occurs in the veins of other vascular beds, particularly in the splanchnic area. This is brought about by contraction of the smooth muscle walls of the capacitance vessels induced by sympathetic stimulation from the circulatory centre and prevents blood pressure falling (part of the pressure receptor reflex). If this counter-regulatory measure fails, the venous return to the heart is no longer sufficient to maintain an adequate cardiac output and blood pressure falls, with orthostatic collapse. Insufficient filling of the capacitance vessels, with resulting hypovolaemia and fall in blood pressure, is to be expected in all conditions which lead to fluid loss from the circulation. These conditions include high-grade burns, intestinal paralysis with fluid accumulation in the atonic region, and fluid loss due to vomiting, diarrhoea or excessive renal excretion.

3.10 PULMONARY CIRCULATION

The vascular resistance in the pulmonary circulation is considerably lower than the peripheral resistance in the systemic circulation. Thus, the right heart has only to maintain a mean pressure of 10–15mmHg in the pulmonary arteries in order to drive the cardiac output through the lung. Only a fraction of the total pulmonary vessels are open at any one time. If cardiac output increases the resistance in the pulmonary circulation can be considerably reduced and a rise in pulmonary artery pressure largely avoided. Perfusion is reduced in less aerated regions of the lungs since the arterioles of the lungs contract (in contrast to those of the systemic circulation) when the oxygen saturation falls and the carbon dioxide saturation rises.

If the pressure in the pulmonary circulation increases and the colloid osmotic pressure of the plasma falls below 25mmHg, there may be an escape of fluid into the pulmonary alveoli (pulmonary oedema). The risk of pulmonary oedema is higher when right ventricular function is intact, and the left ventricle is unable to cope with the preload (diastolic filling), as in acute left ventricular failure or mitral valve stenosis.

4 Examination Methods

4.1 RANGE OF DIAGNOSTIC METHODS

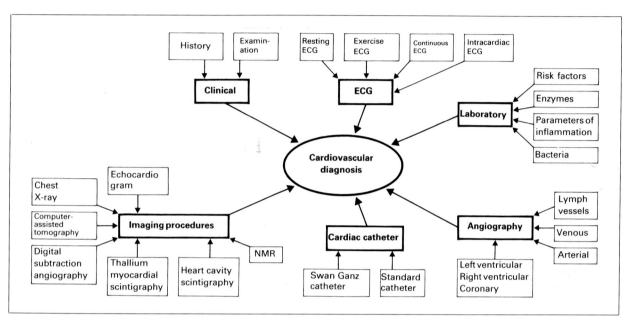

Fig. 4.1 Cardiovascular diagnostic procedure.

The taking of a careful medical history can provide important clues to the diagnosis (Fig. 4.1):

Family history (hypertension, hypercholesterolaemia, coronary heart disease, sudden cardiac death, e.g. hypertrophic cardiomyopathy or long QT syndrome). Personal history of cigarette smoking, hypertension, diabetes mellitus, hypercholesterolaemia, obesity (risk factors for coronary heart disease and peripheral arterial occlusive disease).

Alcohol abuse (alcoholic cardiomyopathy).

Past history of rheumatic fever or scarlet fever (rheumatic valvular heart disease).

Dyspnoea at rest or during exercise, orthopnoea, paroxysmal nocturnal dyspnoea, ankle oedema, dry cough, nocturia (heart failure).

Palpitations, dizziness or loss of consciousness (cardiac arrhythmias).

Exertional chest pain (angina pectoris in coronary heart disease), prolonged rest pain (myocardial infarction, dissecting aortic aneurysm).

The physical examination follows the format of inspection, palpation, percussion and auscultation.

1. Careful inspection can provide important clues to the diagnosis. One should inspect for nutritional status, facial colour (malar flush in mitral stenosis, anaemia, polycythaemia or cyanosis), dyspnoea, abnormal wave form in neck veins or neck arteries, raised jugular venous pressure, peripheral oedema, finger clubbing (congenital cyanotic heart disease), splinter haemorrhages (infective endocarditis), skeletal abnormalities associated with congenital heart disease, e.g. long fingers in Marfan's syndrome.

2. Palpation is used to examine the position and character of the apex beat, abnormal pulsations over the precordium associated with left and right ventricular hypertrophy, and to examine the pulse in various sites (radial, carotid, femoral and dorsalis pedis arteries).

3. Auscultation of the heart provides important information about the quality of the heart sounds, additional heart sounds (third or fourth heart sound in heart failure), systolic murmurs (aortic stenosis, pulmonary stenosis, mitral or tricuspid incompetence, ventricular septal defect), diastolic murmurs (aortic or pulmonary valve incompetence, mitral or tricuspid sten-

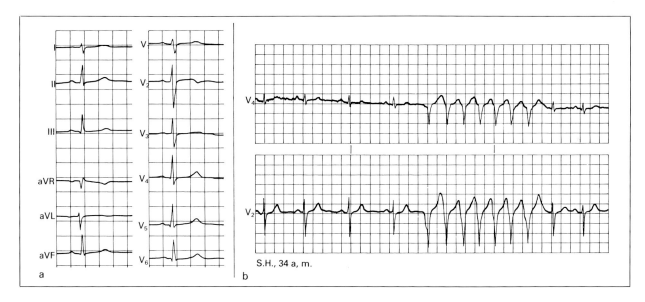

Fig. 4.2 a) Resting ECG. b) Continuous ECG with brief ventricular tachycardia.

osis), continuous murmurs (machinery murmur of persistent ductus arteriosus, arteriovenous fistula).

4. The presence of pulmonary oedema in left ventricular failure can be recognized by the presence of fine crepitations at the lung bases and signs of right ventricular failure include the presence of pitting ankle oedema.

5. Blood pressure is measured separately on both arms using a sphygomanometer cuff. If coarctation of the aorta is suspected, the pressure in both legs should also be recorded (blood pressure lower in legs).

4.2 ELECTROCARDIOGRAM

The electrocardiogram (ECG) is a recording of the changes in surface potential over the atria and ventricles associated with the propagation of electrical impulses (Fig. 4.2). The resulting electric fields spread throughout the entire body, which can be regarded as a volume conductor. Voltage differences can be detected on the skin with suitable surface electrodes and recorded after amplification.

4.2.1 ECG at rest

Several electrode positions are used for recording the surface electrocardiogram: standard leads I, II, III (Einthoven leads), aVR, aVL and aVF (Goldberger leads), and the unipolar chest leads V1–V6 (Wilson's leads). The 12-lead recording makes up the standard electrocardiogram recording, although other lead positions can be used for research purposes. The pattern of deflections from the different lead positions provides information about the electrical axis of the heart, delay or block in conduction through the AV node and His–Purkinje system, enlargement of the atria or hypertrophy of the ventricular myocardium, the presence of myocardial necrosis and arrhythmias. The ECG can provide essential information in patients with coronary heart disease, especially in myocardial infarction, arrhythmias, atrial or ventricular enlargement or hypertrophy, cor pulmonale, pericarditis and electrolyte disturbances.

4.2.2 The exercise ECG

The ECG can be recorded during physical exercise. This usually takes the form of incremental levels of exercise using a bicycle ergometer or continuous belt treadmill system. Various protocols have been devised but usually take the form of 3min of exercise at each stage, with the subject progressing to the next level until the target heart rate or expected level of submaximal work activity has been achieved. The electrocardiogram, heart rate and blood pressure are measured immediately before exercise and at the end of each exercise stage.

In many patients the resting electrocardiogram is normal, but abnormalities are brought out by physical exertion. The following information can be obtained from the exercise ECG:

The physical fitness of the patient.
Blood pressure response to exercise.
The appearance of myocardial ischaemia.
The occurrence of exercise-induced arrhythmias.

The exercise ECG is most commonly used for the diagnosis of functionally significant coronary artery disease. Generally speaking, the earlier that ECG abnormalities reflecting ischaemia develop and the more marked the changes become, the greater the likelihood of severe coronary disease.

4.2.3   Continuous ambulatory ECG monitoring

The ECG can be recorded onto magnetic tape continuously for a 24-hour period using two bipolar chest wall leads, corresponding to leads V2 and V5. The tape is then analysed on an instrument specifically devised for this purpose. The following parameters are of particular interest: minimum, mean and maximum heart rate, prolonged pauses of more than two seconds, supraventricular and ventricular arrhythmias and variations in the ST segment reflecting symptomatic or silent myocardial ischaemia. Twenty-four-hour ECG recording is used to clarify the patient's symptoms (palpitation, dizziness or syncope), and to document intermittent disorders of rate or rhythm which would not normally be picked up on the routine 12-lead ECG. It can also be used to assess the prognosis of the patient with life-threatening arrhythmias and to monitor the effects of anti-arrhythmic treatment.

4.2.4   ECG in coronary heart disease

In ischaemic heart disease, the ECG may be normal or may show signs of previous myocardial infarction in the form of deep, broad Q waves and/or T wave abnormalities. Persistent elevation of the ST segment is a sign of ventricular aneurysm formation.

4.2.5   ECG in acute myocardial infarction

Although the electrocardiogram may remain normal for up to 24h after the onset of acute myocardial infarction, more commonly the ECG shows typical abnormalities within a few hours of acute coronary occlusion which will confirm the diagnosis of a heart attack. Evolution of ECG changes progresses through several stages over a period of days, providing a guide as to whether the infarct is acute, subacute or in the healing stage. Examination of the 12-lead ECG also allows localization of the site of infarction (anterior wall, inferior, inferolateral, anteroseptal, etc).

4.2.6   ECG in other diseases

The ECG can show changes reflecting increased pressure or stress in the right atrium and ventricle which may be caused by valvular defects, atrial septal defects, or conditions causing increased pulmonary vascular resistance. Left atrial enlargement (as occurs in mitral stenosis), causes increased duration of the P wave, whereas right atrial enlargement causes increased amplitude of the P wave. Conditions causing an increased systolic pressure load on the left ventricle (arterial hypertension, aortic stenosis), lead to left ventricular hypertrophy which causes increased amplitude of the QRS complex, often associated with ST segment depression and T wave inversion (left ventricular strain pattern). Extrasystoles (supraventricular or ventricular) may be present on the electrocardiogram in addition to conduction disorders (AV block, left and right bundle branch block) in specific heart muscle diseases, e.g. hypertrophic cardiomyopathy, dilated cardiomyopathy, amyloid.

4.3 IMAGING TECHNIQUES

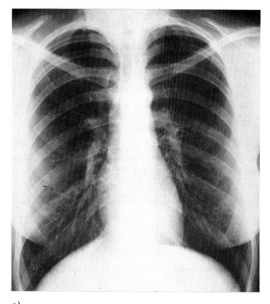
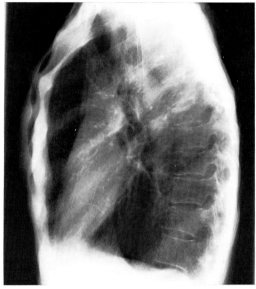

a)

b)

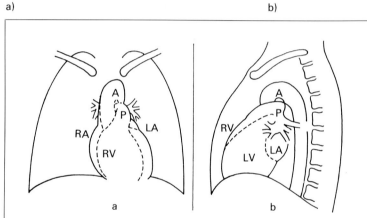

Fig. 4.3 Radiographs of heart and lungs.
a) AP projection. b) Lateral projection.
RA: Right atrium.
LA: Left atrium.
A: Aorta.
P: Pulmonary artery.
RV: Right ventricle.
LV: Left ventricle.

4.3.1 Chest X-ray

The structure of the lungs, heart and mediastinum can be examined with the aid of chest X-rays (Fig. 4.3). Abnormalities of the thoracic skeleton are also of interest, e.g. rib notching in coarctation of the aorta.

A standard chest X-ray provides information about the size and shape of the heart shadow, which is altered in diseased states. In health, the maximum transverse diameter of the heart shadow occupies less than half the transverse diameter off the chest. Enlargement of the heart shadow usually reflects enlargement or dilatation of the left ventricle. The contour of the heart shadow is also altered in disease states, e.g. straightening of the left heart border in mitral stenosis. Alteration in the appearances of the lung fields is seen in the presence of left ventricular failure. The earliest radiological sign of left ventricular failure is upper lobe venous diversion, whereby the pulmonary veins in the upper lung zones become abnormally prominent and dilated. With increasing degrees of vascular congestion, fluid is forced out of the vascular compartment into the interstitial spaces. This is seen as haziness around the bronchi and vessels and in the lung fissures. Engorgement of the lymphatics causes thickening of the interlobular septi, which is best seen in the costophrenic angles as horizontal white lines called Kerley B lines. In severe heart failure there is transudation of oedema fluid into the intra-alveolar spaces causing fluffy white shadows which spread outwards from the hilar areas (bat's wing appearance). In chronic heart failure, with pulmonary hypertension, other changes include the development of pleural effusions, pulmonary haemosiderosis, lung fibrosis, and aneurysmal dilatation of the pulmonary veins.

4.3.2 Computed tomography (CT scanning)

Cross-sectional images of the structures in the thorax can be obtained by the special radiographic technique of CT scanning. A finely collimated X-ray beam is passed through the body and the intensity of the exiting X-rays are picked up by radiation detectors. The X-ray tube is housed in a circular gantry, which is then rotated around the patient. A computer analyzes the intensity of radiation after it has been attenuated by passing through the body from many different angles. The computer generates cross-sectional slices with a spacial and density resolution far greater than that of ultrasound or radionuclide imaging (Fig. 4.4b). Differentiation of structures can be further enhanced by injection of intravenous angiographic contrast media which accentuate the differences between the heart chambers and the cardiac wall. The following information can be obtained:

Cardiac chambers: the size, shape and volume of the cardiac chambers can be accurately measured through multiple CT scan slices taken at different levels through the heart. Intracavity thrombi and mural thrombus can also be identified.

Ventricular musculature: as the myocardium is sharply delineated from the opacified intracavity blood and the radiolucent epicardial fat on the outer surface, accurate measurement of ventricular muscle mass can be obtained. The thickness of myocardium can be examined at multiple levels. The presence of thinning due to myocardial infarction or intramural tumour can be identified.

Pericardium: thickening of the pericardium in constrictive pericarditis, pericardial effusions, tumours or cysts may be seen.

Coronary vessels: calcification of atheromatous plaques in the proximal coronary vessels may be detected as they are relatively stationary, but the tortuous course and motion of the distal coronary vessels make this an unsuitable technique for assessment of coronary disease.

Coronary artery bypass grafts: the proximal ends of aortocoronary venous bypass grafts can be identified after injection of contrast material.

Congenital heart disease: the transverse slices produced by CT scanning are not always the optimal technique for visualization of congenital lesions. However, shunts can be identified by taking multiple CT scans after intravenous injection of angiographic contrast material. Some structural abnormalities can be readily detected.

Aorta: serial CT scans allow accurate measurement of the width of the aorta and the presence of aortic aneurysm. In dissection of the aorta, the intimal flap may be identified particularly after injection of contrast material.

4.3.3 Digital subtraction angiography

This technique involves conversion of the X-ray image intensifier fluoroscopic picture into a digital signal to be analyzed by a computer system. The improved contrast definition obtained by digital subtraction angiography is useful in the following situations:

Pulmonary angiography: to identify pulmonary embolism, vascular malformations and arteriovenous fistula.
Cardiac chambers: computer programs can be used to provide wall enhancement, regional or global wall motion or ejection fraction. Selective enhancement of regions of interest can assist with the detection of tumours or thrombi and the assessment of congenital or acquired heart defects, with or without valve involvement.
Major blood vessels: digital subtraction angiography can be applied to imaging of the major vessels of the thorax, neck, abdomen, pelvis, thigh and calf.

4.3.4 Echocardiography

This is a non-invasive method of imaging the heart using ultrasound waves. It provides detailed information on cardiac structure and is a first-line investigation in many forms of heart disease (Fig. 4.4a). Its uses include:

Clarification of cardiac anatomy (acquired or congenital heart defects). Valve function (valvular stenosis, prolapse, vegetations in infective endocarditis).
Left ventricular wall thickness (hypertension, hypertrophic obstructive cardiomyopathy).
Ventricular function (left or right ventricular dilatation, regional hypokinesis, left ventricular aneurysm, generalized hypokinesis in dilated cardiomyopathy).

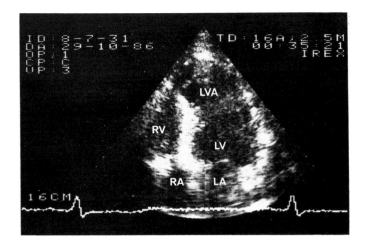

a) Echocardiogram.

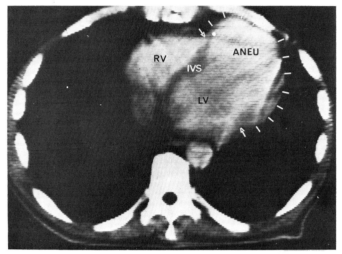

b) Computerized tomogram.

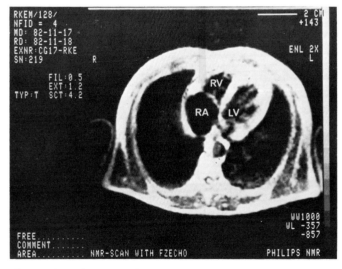

c) NMR image of the heart.

Fig. 4.4 Imaging procedures.

Intracavity abnormalities (left or right atrial myxoma, mural thrombus).
Pericardial diseases (pericardial effusion, tumour).
Prosthetic valves (assessment of valve opening).
Aortic root (aneurysm formation, aortic dissection).

The ultrasound image of the heart can only be obtained at sites where the lungs are not covering the heart. Two 'windows' are commonly used in the echocardiogram examination at the left sternal edge in the third or fourth interspace and at the cardiac apex. The quality of the picture obtained is adversely affected by obesity, by pulmonary emphysema, chest deformities or by assisted ventilation. The ultrasound beam can be angled to provide several cross-sectional images of the heart in different planes. Routinely, the echocardiogram will include measurements of the dimensions of the left atrium, left and right ventricles, aortic root and ventricular septal thickness. The motion of the mitral, aortic and tricuspid valves is also assessed, although the pulmonary valve is less frequently seen.

4.3.5   Nuclear cardiology

Radioisotopes can be used in the assessment of patients with cardiac disease. Thallium scanning is useful in the assessment of myocardial perfusion, and technetium scanning for left and right ventricular function.

Thallium scanning

This technique is used to detect diffuse or regional myocardial ischaemia. It can also differentiate between a reversible ischaemic defect and a persistent defect which usually indicates previous myocardial infarction. Thallium scanning is particularly useful in patients who have symptoms of angina but in whom exercise ECG testing is contra-indicated, or the patient is unable to exercise adequately, or the results of exercise testing were equivocal. It can also be used to assess the haemodynamic significance of a coronary stenosis found at coronary arteriography.

After radiolabelled thallium-201 is injected intravenously, it is extracted by the myocardium and stored intracellularly against a gradient. The distribution of thallium in the myocardium depends on regional blood flow. Cells damaged by hypoxia can no longer accumulate thallium against a gradient, or lose intracellularly stored thallium to the interstitium. Thallium distribution within the myocardium is recorded by a gamma camera and processed to produce an image. The distribution of thallium can be assessed both during exercise and two hours after resting. In a patient who has a functionally significant coronary stenosis, a perfusion defect will be seen on the stress image, but the image taken in the recovery phase will be normal, indicating that viable myocardial tissue is still present which only becomes ischaemic during exercise. This phenomenon is called redistribution. Diffuse thallium perfusion defects are seen in

patients with cardiomyopathy, severe multi-vessel coronary disease or patients with microvascular coronary disease.

As an alternative to exercise stress testing for thallium imaging, pharmacological stress can be applied. The agent used is dipyridamole, which is injected intravenously and produces maximal coronary vasodilatation. If a functionally significant coronary stenosis is present, there will be a relative underperfusion of the area subtended by that artery producing a perfusion defect on the scan.

Radionuclide ventriculography

Regional and global contractile function of the left and right ventricles can be assessed by technetium scanning. The initial bolus of technetium can be followed in its passage through the left and right heart. As there is a temporal and anatomical separation of radioactivity within each cardiac chamber, the function of both left and right ventricles can be assessed from a single injection. Furthermore, the temporal separation allows identification of intra-cardiac shunts, whereby radioactive counts may appear early in the left side of the heart, or a double peak in the pulmonary circulation may be present due to recirculation from left-to-right shunting. A computer can be used to trace the outlines of the left and right ventricle chambers and analyze regional and global wall motion, as well as detecting the presence of left ventricular or aortic arch aneurysm.

4.3.6   NMR tomography (nuclear spin tomography)

The latest method for non-invasive evaluation of the heart is nuclear magnetic resonance imaging (Fig. 4.4c). Two- and three-dimensional images of the structures in the path of the electromagnetic field can be created with the aid of a computer program. It produces high resolution images which can be used in the following:

All aspects of the anatomy of the heart and major blood vessels, including assessment of congenital heart disease, shunt identification, valve areas and valvular incompetence.
Myocardial abnormalities (site and extent of infarction, viable myocardium versus scar tissue).
Cardiac masses (intracavity thrombus, myocardial tumours).
Pericardial disease (thickened pericardium, effusion volume, transudate versus exudate).
Ventricular function (contractility, three-dimensional imaging of shape and volume).

4.4 CARDIAC CATHETERIZATION

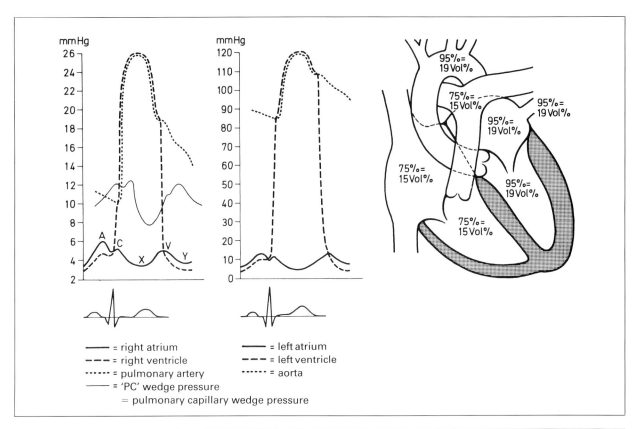

= right atrium
= right ventricle
= pulmonary artery
= 'PC' wedge pressure
= pulmonary capillary wedge pressure

= left atrium
= left ventricle
= aorta

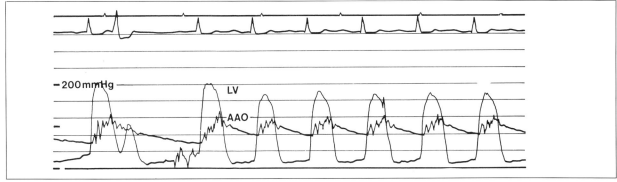

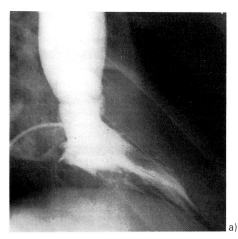

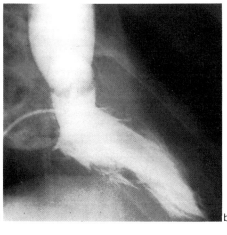

Fig. 4.5 Scheme of cardiac catheterization studies.
a) Aortic valve stenosis, pressure curve.
b) Aortic valve stenosis, laevocardiogram.

4.4.1 Catheterization procedures

This is undertaken to study intracardiac pressures and haemodynamics, left ventricular function and to visualize the coronary arteries. Two principal catheterization procedures are used:

1. Swan-Ganz catheterization. A thin, multi-lumen catheter is inserted into either an antecubital vein or a central vein (subclvian, internal jugular) and advanced to the right atrium. Right atrial pressure is recorded and then a balloon at the tip of the catheter is inflated to facilitate passage of the catheter through the tricuspid valve with the blood flow into the right ventricle, where pressures are again recorded before advancement of the catheter through the pulmonary vein to the main pulmonary artery. When the catheter is pushed further out into a distal pulmonary arterial branch, the inflated balloon completely occludes the lumen. At that point, the pressure recording changes from a pulmonary arterial wave form to that of left atrial pressure which is transmitted backwards through the pulmonary veins and capillary network. Thus, the pulmonary occluded pressure or 'wedge pressure' is an indirect measurement of left atrial and left ventricular end-diastolic pressure. Cardiac output can be measured directly by a cold dilution procedure (thermodilution). A known volume of ice-cold saline is injected as a bolus into the right atrium through one port in the side wall of the Swan-Ganz catheter, and the change in temperature is noted at the tip of the catheter in the pulmonary artery by a temperature thermistor. A computer analyzes the change in temperature, together with the time taken for the bolus of cold saline to reach the pulmonary artery in order to calculate cardiac output. Swan-Ganz catheterization can be carried out as a bedside technique without X-ray screening and is useful in the coronary care or intensive care setting to assess circulatory haemodynamics after acute myocardial infarction or in patients who are in shock. Systemic and pulmonary vascular resistance can be calculated from the cardiac output, intracardiac pressures and mean systemic arterial pressure. Knowledge of these measurements is useful to optimize therapeutic interventions aimed at restoring circulatory haemodynamics to normal.
2. In full cardiac catheterization, catheters are introduced both into the right and left sides of the heart to measure pressure in all four cardiac chambers. By simultaneously measuring the pulmonary occluded pressure from the right heart catheter, and the left ventricular end-diastolic pressure from the left heart catheter, the transmitral valve gradient can be measured. Oxygen saturations can be measured in different parts of the heart to evaluate and quantify abnormal communications in the heart (atrial septal defect, ventricular septal defect, patent ductus arteriosus, aortopulmonary shunts). Angiographic contrast media can be injected through the catheters to visualize the cardiac chambers and the X-ray images are recorded on cine film for later analysis. Similarly, the coronary arteries can be selectively cannulated and after injection of a small volume of contrast medium, the images are recorded on film. Injections are repeated in several X-ray projection angles for full visualization of the coronary vasculature. In this way, localized constrictions or occlusions of the vessels can be documented.

Left ventricular angiography is the gold standard for assessing left ventricular pump function. It gives an estimate of global and regional left ventricular function and ejection fraction can be calculated from the formula end-diastolic volume minus end-systolic volume, divided by end-diastolic volume and multiplied by 100 (expressed as a percentage).

4.4.2 Selective angiography

By selecting suitable preformed catheters, the left and right coronary arteries can be selectively cannulated and the vessels imaged with contrast medium and recorded on film. A wide range of catheters have been designed for selective injection into other peripheral vessels to assess the presence of stenoses or occlusions (e.g. carotid arteries, renal arteries, iliac and femoral arteries). This angiographic procedure is a prerequisite for choosing the most appropriate therapeutic intervention, e.g. transluminal catheter dilatation, surgery).

4.4.3 Lymphangiography

In the same way, the lymphatic vessels can be filled with contrast medium and radiographically visualized (lymphangiography). This reveals the lymph vessels of the lower limbs and pelvis (abnormalities, dilatations, rarefaction) and, 24h later, the lymph nodes of the pelvis and abdomen will become opacified (imaging of primary and secondary lymph node tumours).

4.5 POST-MORTEM CORONARY ANGIOGRAPHY

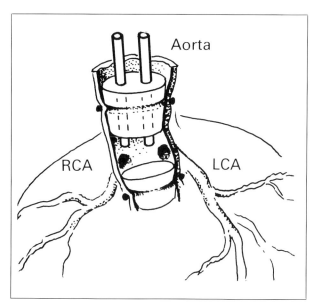

Fig. 4.6 Diagram of heart prepared for the contrast medium technique. Aortic root blocked with wedges below and above the coronary arteries (RCA: right coronary artery; LCA: left coronary artery).

Fig. 4.7 Angiogram of an unexcised post-mortem heart in the usual projection.
1: Main trunk of right coronary artery with vascular lumen blocked by a thrombus (arrow).
2: Left circumflex branch.
3: Anterior interventricular branch.
4: Posterior interventricular branch. Wall irregularities caused by arteriosclerosis in practically all major vascular branches. Right supply type.

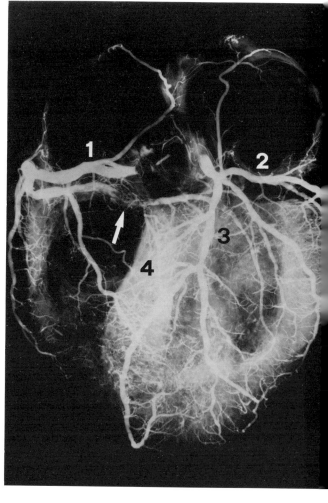

Post-mortem angiograms of the coronary system had been possible (Baumgarten, 1899) long before the technological advancements for coronary arteriography on live subjects had been achieved. The pathologist now uses techniques which allow a simple comparison of post-mortem and radiographic findings with angiograms taken in life. In this procedure, contrast medium is injected down the coronary arteries via the 'natural route', after sealing the aortic root above and below the coronary ostia. All the vessels emerging from this region are visualized, including bypass grafts. The coronary ostia are also well seen.

The X-ray projections of post-mortem coronary angiogram in the undissected heart usually show the organ lying on its posterior wall. This view of the coronary system is not normally obtained by angiograms in life and thus not familiar to the clinical cardiologist. Post-mortem coronary angiograms taken in the planes normally used in the cardiac catheterization laboratory (right anterior oblique, left anterior oblique), (Fig. 4.8) promote understanding between cardiologists and pathologists. Pre- and post-mortem coronary angiograms can also be compared in the same patient, which may help with the understanding of changes in atheroma with time or the fate of thrombi.

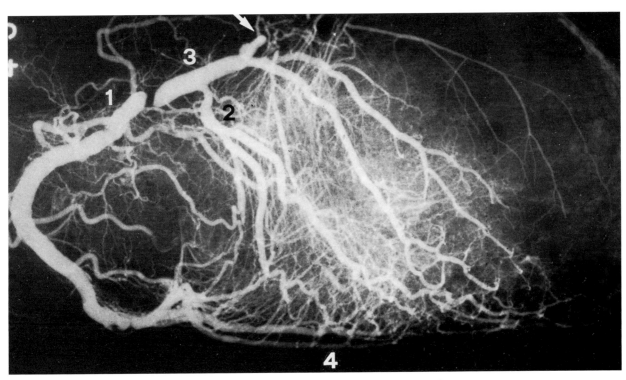

Fig. 4.8 Post-mortem coronary angiogram in projection corresponding to RAO.
1: Main trunk of right coronary artery.
2: Left circumflex branch.
3: Anterior interventricular branch with interruption (arrow).
4: Posterior interventricular branch. Enormous true aneurysm of left ventricular wall.

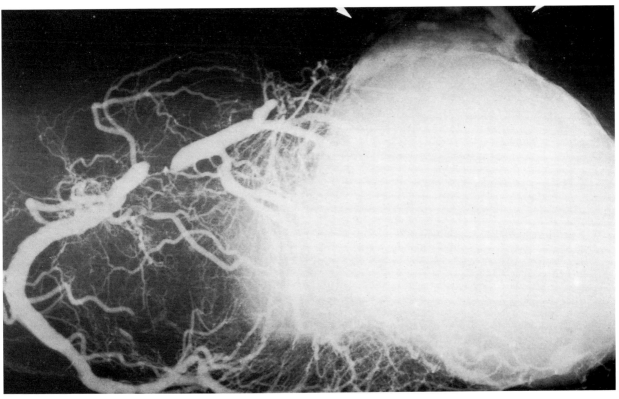

Fig. 4.9 Image as in Fig. 4.8 after additional filling of left ventricle with contrast medium (ventriculography).

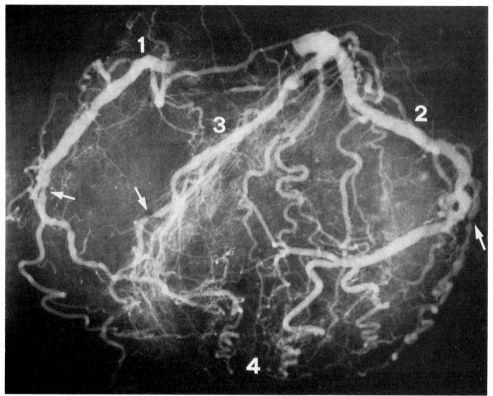

Fig. 4.10 Post-mortem coronary angiogram in projection corresponding to LAO.
1: Main trunk of right coronary artery.
2: Left circumflex branch.
3: Anterior interventricular branch.
4: Posterior interventricular branch. Multiple and, in parts, relatively broad, peripherally located constrictions of the lumen of numerous large vascular branches (arrows).

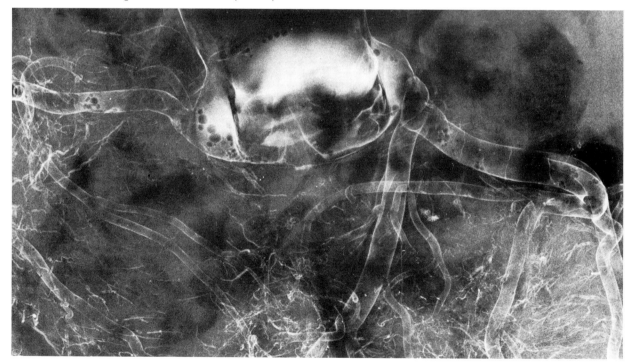

Fig. 4.11 Post-mortem coronary angiogram by the double contrast method with imaging of the coronary ostia.
Projection as in Fig. 4.10. Vessels free from atherosclerosis. 75 mm Hg gas pressure.

5 Variations in the Shape and Size of the Heart

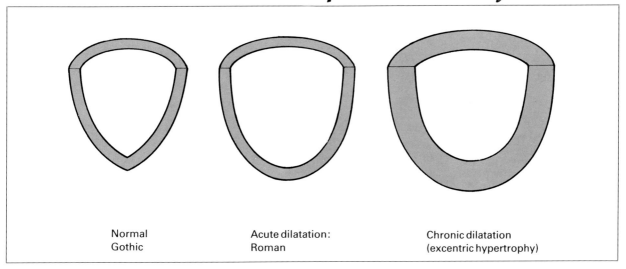

Normal
Gothic

Acute dilatation:
Roman

Chronic dilatation
(excentric hypertrophy)

Fig. 5.1 Shape of left ventricular lumen.

Changes in the shape and size of the heart can be examined in post-mortem specimens and described in terms of weight, wall thickness and volume of the heart. In life, echocardiography provides a useful tool for studying alterations in wall thickness and chamber size (Fig. 5.1).

1. Weight: the weight of the heart depends mainly on age, body weight and physiological loading conditions. The greatest weights (up to 500g) in health are found in those who undergo strenuous physical exertion (athlete's heart).
2. Wall thickness: increase in the wall thickness or hypertrophy predominantly affects the ventricular walls and is an indication of an abnormal chronic stress imposed upon that chamber (e.g. hypertension, aortic stenosis).
3. Heart volume: the size of the heart depends on its muscular mass (hypertrophy or atrophy) and the volumes of the cardiac chambers. In autopsy specimens, only approximate values can be obtained since they depend on the degree of myocardial contraction. Post-mortem ventricular volumes are 10–25ml, though they can be much higher in patients with dilated cardiomyopathy.

On the basis of the parameters weight, ventricular wall thickness and ventricular volume, the following abnormalities can be described.

5.1 CARDIAC HYPERTROPHY

5.1.1 Concentric cardiac hypertrophy

An increase in mass of one or both ventricles occurs as a result of chronic pressure overload. The most common causes are hypertension and aortic valve stenosis. Concentric right ventricular hypertrophy is called cor pulmonale, and is due to pulmonary hypertension induced by primary lung disease. Right ventricular hypertrophy also occurs in pulmonary hypertension secondary to left ventricular failure, mitral stenosis or congenital heart disease, but is excluded from the definition of cor pulmonale. Morphologically, there is a marked increase in weight of the ventricles (extreme form; cor bovinum with a weight of 800g or more). In left ventricular hypertrophy a cross-section of the apex reveals a markedly thickened wall (up to 20mm) and a circular small lumen. The right ventricular wall is much thinner than that of the left ventricle and a thickness of 6–8mm is consistent with a severe degree of hypertrophy. The endocardial surface of the right ventricle is trabeculated and this becomes particularly striking in right ventricular hypertrophy.

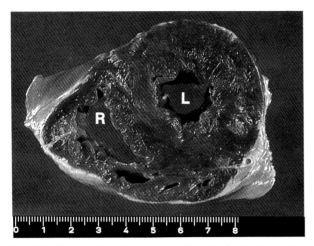

Fig. 5.2 Normal heart. Cross-section through the right (R) and left (L) ventricles.

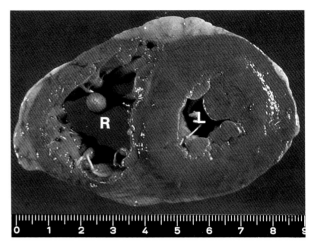

Fig. 5.3 Concentric hypertrophy of left ventricular wall.

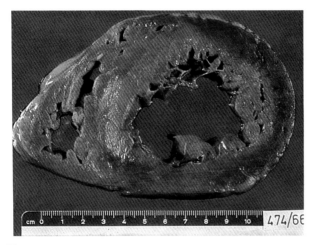

Fig. 5.4 Eccentric hypertrophy of left ventricular wall.

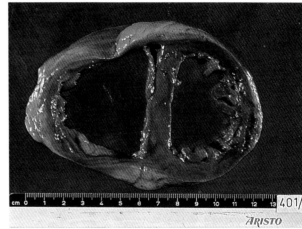

Fig. 5.5 Global dilatation.

5.1.2 Asymmetric cardiac hypertrophy

This can be due to a primary cardiomyopathy of either ventricle but also occurs as a result of volume overload as a result of valvular heart disease. Macroscopically, the heart is enlarged and heavy with a rounded apex whose lumen is broadened in cross-section. Histologically, the hypertrophy of myocardial fibres is best seen in cross-section. The myocytes are broad, with misshapen nuclei, and in longitudinal section, the nuclei are large, barrel-shaped and hyperchromatic.

5.2 CARDIAC DILATATION

Dilatation of the cardiac chambers is usually associated with only a moderate degree of wall hypertrophy and the total heart weight is only slightly increased. Dilatation of a cardiac chamber is a response to volume overload, as may occur with aortic or mitral incompetence, or as a result of loss of contractile function, e.g. acute myocardial infarction.

5.3   CARDIAC ATROPHY

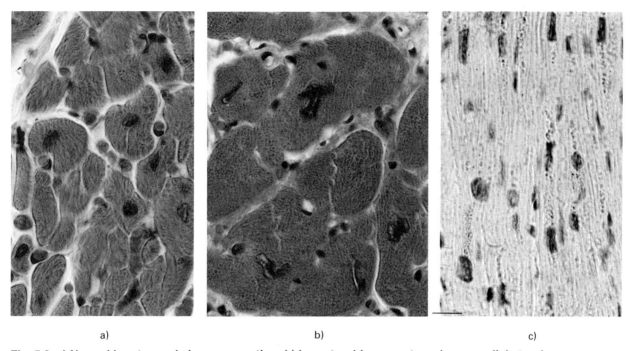

a)   b)   c)

Fig. 5.6 a) Normal heart muscle in cross-section; b) hypertrophic myocytes; c) myocardial atrophy.
Myocytes in longitudinal section (stained only with haematoxylin). Profuse lipofuscin pigment close to the nucleus.

In cardiac atrophy, the weight of the heart is subnormal (less than 250g). It is particularly common in cachexia associated with loss of subepicardial fatty tissue and the coronary arteries (Fig. 5.7) are seen to have a tortuous course. In open section, the myocardium appears dark brown due to myocytic lipofuscinosis. Even a hypertrophic heart may show evidence of atrophy at the same time, so that the weight of the heart cannot be used as a guide as to the presence of atrophy. In some individuals, the heart undergoes progressive loss of muscle mass known as involution of the heart or senile cardiomyopathy. In others, a progressive increase in wall thickness occurs with increasing age, possibly as a result of loss of elasticity and compliance in the aorta, causing systolic hypertension.

5.3.1   Polyploidization

The DNA content of the myocardial nucleus depends on age and cardiac function. Up to the age of 12 years, the nucleus is diploid while in adults it is predominantly tetraploid. When excessive loading conditions are imposed upon the heart, there is polyploidization, i.e. the DNA content increases.

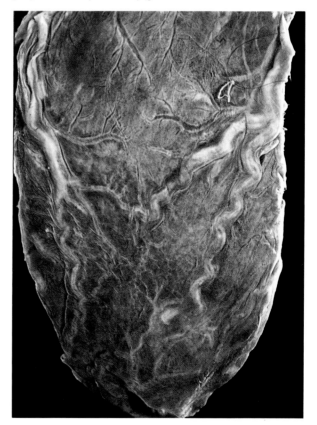

Fig. 5.7 Cardiac atrophy. Disappearance of subepicardial fatty tissues and convoluted course of the coronary arteries.

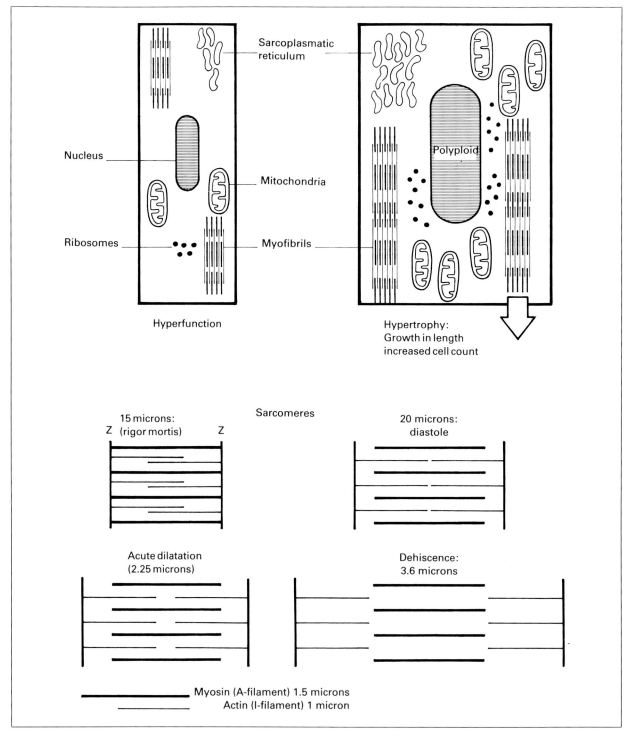

Fig. 5.8 Ultrastructure of myocytes in cases of hyperfunction, hypertrophy and dilatation.

5.3.2 Electron microscopy (Fig. 5.8)

In myocardial hypertrophy, the individual myocytes are enlarged, while the elementary fibrils are more numerous, but not broader. The number of mitochondria also increases. Rough endoplastic reticulum, lipofuscin granules and newly formed myofibrils (lacking sarcomeres) are found in the nuclear region. The cell nucleus and nucleolus are enlarged and the cell boundaries appear convoluted.

6 Cardiovascular Diseases

6.1 HEART FAILURE

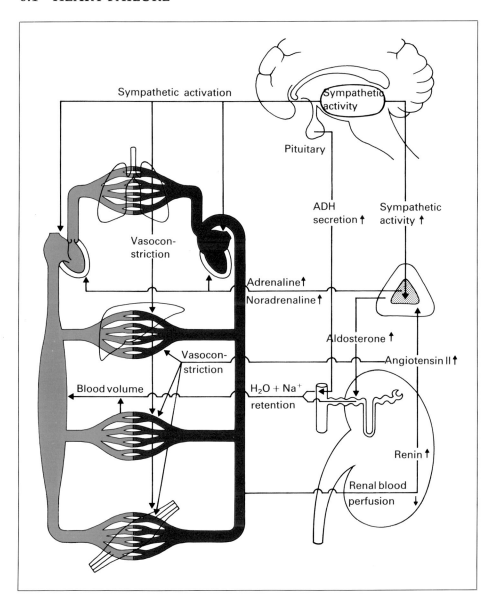

Sympathetic activation

Sympathetic activity

Pituitary

ADH secretion ↑

Sympathetic activity ↑

Vasocon- striction

Adrenaline ↑

Noradrenaline ↑

Aldosterone ↑

Vasocon- striction

Angiotensin II ↑

Blood volume

$H_2O + Na^+$ retention

Renin ↑

Renal blood perfusion ↓

Fig. 6.1 Heart failure.

Definition: heart failure is a clinical state due to the inability of the heart to maintain a circulating blood volume adequate for the metabolic requirements of the body despite sufficient venous return (Fig. 6.1).

Aetiology: the causes of heart failure are:

1. Impaired myocardial contractility, e.g. myocardial infarction, cardiomyopathy, myocarditis, metabolic heart disease, endocrine heart disease, drugs such as beta blockers, and anti-arrhythmic agents.
2. Volume overload, e.g. aortic regurgitation, mitral regurgitation.
3. Pressure overload, e.g. aortic stenosis, hypertension.
4. Impaired left ventricular filling, e.g. severe mitral stenosis, restrictive cardiomyopathy, constrictive pericarditis, pericardial effusion.
5. Arrhythmias

Pathophysiology

Heart failure may be due to either failure of the left ventricle or the right ventricle, or both ventricles (biventricular failure). Left ventricular failure causes congestion in the pulmonary circulation, whereas right ventricular failure causes peripheral venous congestion. Biventricular failure results in both pulmonary and peripheral congestion. In heart failure, several compensatory mechanisms, which can be either cardiac or extra-cardiac, are stimulated to try to improve cardiac output. The compensatory cardiac mechanisms which can be invoked are an increased heart rate, ventricular hypertrophy or dilatation. The extra-cardiac compensatory mechanisms are activation of the neuro-endocrine system, increased peripheral resistance and redistribution of fluid within the circulation. In heart failure, the neuro-endocrine systems activated are:

1. Increased sympathetic activity
   Reduced cardiac output causes a fall in blood pressure. This stimulates the sympathetic nervous system to produce catecholamines which, in turn, increases the heart rate, myocardial contractility and causes vasoconstriction in an attempt to raise the blood pressure. Blood flow to the kidney, liver and gastro-intestinal tract is reduced.
2. Renin–angiotensin–aldosterone system
   Reduced renal blood flow stimulates the release of renin and aldosterone. Increased renin levels stimulate the production of angiotensin I, which is converted to angiotensin II. This is a potent vasoconstrictor. The increased levels of aldosterone stimulate sodium and water retention by the kidney. The compensatory activation of the neuro-endocrine system in heart failure has both beneficial and deleterious effects on the circulation. The beneficial effects due to activation of the neuro-endocrine system include a rise in blood pressure and increased chronotropic and inotropic effects on the heart. The deleterious effects are increased peripheral resistance and impaired renal perfusion which results in fluid overload.

Symptoms

The symptoms that patients with left ventricular failure may complain of include breathlessness, which may manifest as exertional dyspnoea, orthopnoea or paroxysmal nocturnal dyspnoea. Patients may also complain of chronic fatigue,

muscle weakness or dizziness on exertion. Patients with right ventricular failure may complain of ankle oedema, abdominal distension or upper abdominal pain due to hepatic congestion.

Heart failure is classified into four different functional classes.

New York Heart Association classification of heart failure

Class I
Patients with heart disease but have no limitation of physical activity.
Class II
Patients with heart disease but have slight limitation of physical activity.
Class III
Patients with heart disease who have marked limitation of physical activity.
Class IV
Patients with heart disease who are unable to perform any physical activity due to dyspnoea.

Physical examination

On clinical examination, the patient may be breathless at rest, cyanosed, peripherally shut down with pale, cool peripheries. In predominant left ventricular failure, pulmonary congestion is detected as crepitations and/or pleural effusion. The clinical signs of right ventricular failure include a raised jugular venous pressure, peripheral oedema and hepatomegaly. On auscultation of the heart, cardiac murmurs, third or fourth heart sounds may be heard. The blood pressure may be raised, normal or low, depending on aetiology of the congestive heart failure. The findings on examination of a patient's pulse are also dependent on the aetiology of the patient's congestive heart failure.

Electrocardiogram

Congestive heart failure itself does not have any specific ECG changes. However, the ECG is useful, as it gives information about the cardiac rhythm, ventricular hypertrophy and possible aetiologies of the patient's congestive heart failure, e.g. pathological Q waves are seen in patients who have had myocardial infarcts.

Chest X-ray

The chest X-ray demonstrates the total cardiac size and also if any particular cardiac chamber is enlarged. Evidence of pulmonary congestion, prim-

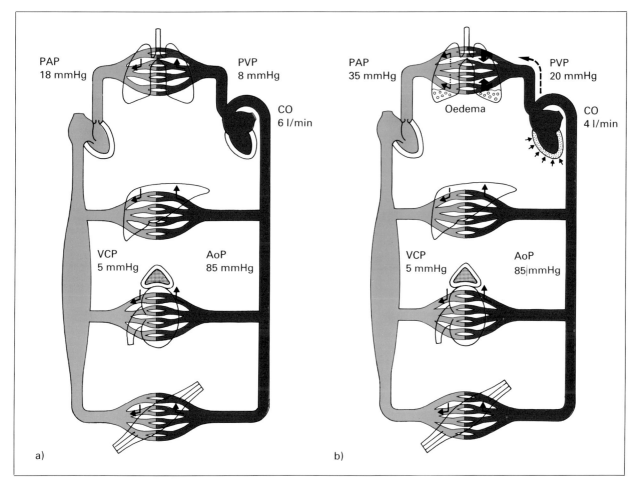

Fig. 6.2 Left ventricular failure. a) Normal. b) Left heart failure. (PAP: pulmonary artery pressure; PVP: pulmonary venous pressure; CO: cardiac output; AoP: aortic pressure; VCP: vena caval pressure.)

ary pulmonary disease and thoracic cage abnormalities may also be seen on the chest X-ray.

Echocardiogram

The echocardiogram can assess non-invasively cardiac chamber size, cardiac valvular abnormalities, contractility of the myocardium with the presence or absence of pericardial effusion.

Nuclear cardiology

Technetium scans can be used to assess ventricular function. Thallium scans can be used to assess myocardial perfusion and are used to help diagnose the cause of congestive heart failure.

Cardiac catheterization

Cardiac catheterization can be used to measure intra-cardiac pressures, blood oxygen saturation in different cardiac chambers and cardiac output.

Cardiac catheterization can also be used to obtain diagnostic myocardial biopsies. Coronary angiography is also performed to assess the state of the patient's coronary arteries.

Dynamic electrocardiography

This may be used to diagnose transient arrhythmias, myocardial ischaemia or investigate pacemaker function in patients with congestive heart failure.

6.1.1 Left ventricular failure

Left ventricular failure is characterized by congestion of the pulmonary circulation as a result of impaired left ventricular performance. The congestion of the pulmonary circulation increases the pulmonary capillary pressure, and if this exceeds plasma oncotic pressure, transudation of fluid occurs and pulmonary oedema develops (Fig. 6.2).

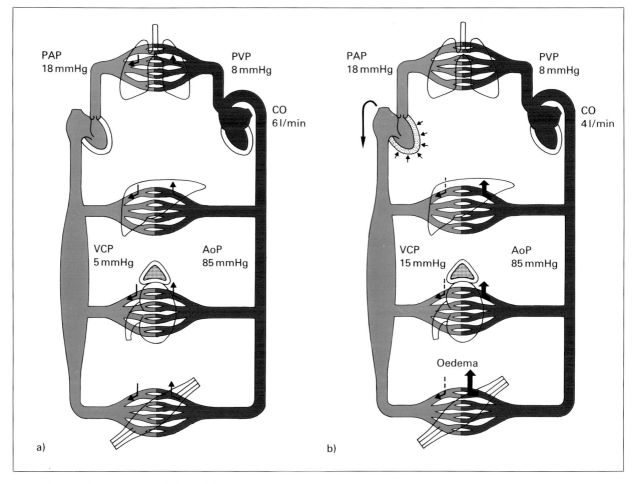

Fig. 6.3 Right heart failure. a) Normal. b) Right heart failure. (PAP: pulmonary artery pressure; PVP: pulmonary venous pressure; CO: cardiac output; AoP: aortic pressure; VCP: vena caval pressure.)

Pulmonary oedema impairs gaseous exchange in the lungs, increases the resistance to air flow in and out of the lungs and reduces pulmonary elasticity. These effects combine to produce hypoxia and an increased workload to breath. Pulmonary oedema is most commonly secondary to left ventricular failure or mitral valve disease. There are also non-cardiac causes of pulmonary oedema, such as hypervolaemia, inhalation of irritant gases, ingested toxins such as paraquat, pulmonary emboli, CNS injury, severe pneumonia or narcotic overdosage.

Symptoms

Patients with acute pulmonary oedema are tachypnoeic and may describe expectoration of pink, frothy sputum. The patient is usually anxious, pale, sweaty and may be cyanosed. On examination of the patient, pulmonary crepitations or rhonchi may be heard, and on auscultation of the heart a third heart sound may be present.

6.1.2   Right ventricular failure

Right ventricular failure causes venous congestion (Fig. 6.3). This results in hepatomegaly, splenomegaly, a raised jugular venous pressure and functional disorders of all the abdominal organs, e.g. abnormal liver function tests, disturbance of gastric absorption and functional renal disorders, with proteinuria and ascites. Right ventricular failure is much less common than left ventricular failure.

Pathogenesis

The causes of right ventricular failure are congenital or acquired disorders of left ventricular function with resultant right ventricular overload and subsequent decompensation, long-standing left-to-right intra-cardiac shunts with secondary pulmonary hypertension, primary valve defects on the right side of the heart, e.g. pulmonary valve stenosis or regurgitation, tricuspid regurgitation, as well as

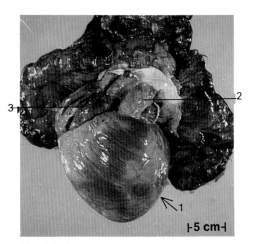

Fig. 6.4 Cor pulmonale.
Marked hypertrophy of the right ventricular wall. Apex of
heart (arrow 1) displaced to the left. (2) Pulmonary artery.
(3) Ascending aorta.

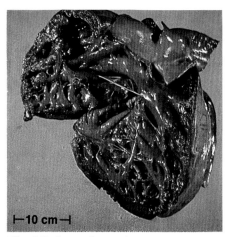

Fig. 6.5 Cor pulmonale.
Section through right ventricle with marked wall thickening
and hypertrophy of trabecular musculature.

rare muscle disorders that predominantly affect the
right ventricle, e.g. arrhythmogenic right ventricular dysplasia. Right ventricular failure can also
occur following inferior myocardial infarct.

6.1.3 Cor pulmonale

Cor pulmonale is defined as hypertrophy of the
right ventricle from diseases affecting the function
and/or structure of the lungs, except when the
pulmonary changes result from disease primarily
affecting the left side of the heart.

Acute cor pulmonale

Acute cor pulmonale is most commonly due to
pulmonary thromboembolism but can also rarely be
due to emboli associated with amniotic fluid, air or
bone marrow post trauma. The embolus obstructs
the pulmonary circulation, impairing the right
ventricular output. The patient may present with a
cardiac arrest following a massive pulmonary
embolus or the patient may complain of dyspnoea,
chest pain, cough with or without haemoptysis. On
examination, the patient will be tachypnoeic,
sweating, cyanosed and may have a raised temperature. The patient will have a tachycardia and, on
auscultation of the heart, a loud P2 will be heard
with third or fourth heart sounds. The JVP will be
raised and crepitations may be heard on auscultation of the chest. Examination of the legs in patients
who have sustained a pulmonary embolus will
reveal clinical evidence of a DVT in only one-third
of these patients. Small pulmonary emboli may not
cause significant haemodynamic disturbance and
present with transient dyspnoea, cough with a

raised temperature and transient cardiac rhythm
disturbance.

Investigation in acute pulmonary embolism

ECG
The changes are not specific for pulmonary embolism and may be transient. Acute right ventricular
strain shows S.I, Q.III, T.III pattern, with anterior T
wave inversion and right bundle branch block.
Right axis deviation or arrhythmias may also occur.

Arterial blood gases
The PaO_2 is usually less than 80mmHg.

Chest X-ray
Patients with small pulmonary emboli may not
have any chest X-ray changes. If the acute pulmonary embolus is large, areas of pulmonary oligaemia,
elevation of a hemidiaphragm, or an enlarged
pulmonary artery may be seen.

Ventilation/perfusion scan
This is a commonly used investigation in the
diagnosis of pulmonary embolism and is a non-
invasive test. Large aggregates of albumin labelled
with technetium are injected intravenously. These
lodge in the pulmonary capillaries. The patient's
chest is then scanned with a gamma camera from a
number of different angles. If a pulmonary embolus
is present, it will cause a defect in the perfusion
scan. Abnormal perfusion scans may also be caused
by other disorders, such as pneumonia, pleural
effusion and asthma. The patient then has a ventilation scan performed. The patient breathes in and
out radioactive xenon 133, while the gamma

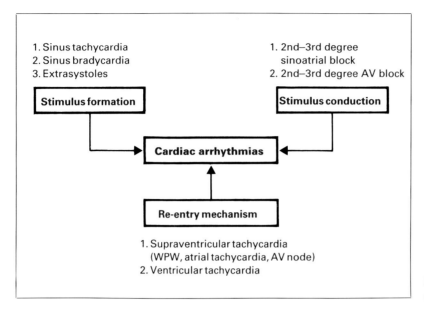

Fig. 6.6 Pathogenesis of cardiac arrhythmias.

camera records its distribution throughout the lungs. If a pulmonary embolus has occurred, the ventilation part of the scan should be normal, whilst the perfusion part is abnormal. Primary pulmonary disease can cause abnormal ventilation scans. Thus, pulmonary emboli cause a ventilation perfusion scan mismatch.

Pulmonary angiography
This is an invasive investigation, in which radiographic contrast is injected into the pulmonary artery. If a pulmonary embolus is obstructing the artery, filling defects are seen.

Predisposing factors
Pulmonary embolism is a common condition and factors predisposing to pulmonary emboli are:

1. Recent surgery or trauma.
2. Prolonged bed rest.
3. Acute myocardial infarction.
4. Malignancy.
5. Congestive heart failure.
6. Previous history of DVT or pulmonary emboli.
7. Polycythaemia.
8. Pelvic inflammatory disease.

Chronic cor pulmonale

Chronic cor pulmonale is observed in:

1. Primary pulmonary parenchymal diseases, e.g. chronic bronchitis, bronchiectasis, chronic asthma, emphysema or pulmonary fibrosis.

2. Disorders of thoracic cage movement, e.g. kyphoscoliosis, obesity and neuromuscular disease.
3. Primary pulmonary vascular disease, e.g. recurrent pulmonary emboli, primary pulmonary hypertension and sickle cell disease.

The patient may complain of dyspnoea, wheeze, lethargy, chest pain, palpitations and cough. The ECG may show features of right ventricular hypertrophy, right axis deviation, P pulmonale, conduction abnormalities and T wave inversion in the right precordial leads. The chest X-ray may show evidence of the underlying cause of cor pulmonale. The right ventricle will be enlarged, with prominent pulmonary arteries and peripheral pruning of the pulmonary vessels. The arterial blood gases depend on the aetiology of the chronic cor pulmonale. The $PaCO_2$ may be elevated in chronic bronchitis or reduced in pulmonary fibrosis. The PaO_2 is usually reduced.

6.2 CARDIAC ARRHYTHMIAS

6.2.1 Definition

These are modifications of the regular heartbeat caused by a number of cardiac and non-cardiac diseases.

Cardiac arrhythmias may cause palpitations, dizziness, loss of consciousness, chest pain and symptoms of heart failure.

The pacemaker cells of the sinoatrial node create the primary electrical impulse. This impulse spreads through the atrial muscle. The impulse then reaches an area of specialized conducting tissue in the right atrium called the AV node. The impulse then passes through this node and down the Bundle of His, bundle branches and through the Purkinje fibres, eventually reaching the ventricular muscle.

6.2.2 Arrhythmias

Sinus bradycardia

Sinus bradycardia is due to the SA node discharging at a rate of less than 60/min. It can be associated with athletic training, increased vagal tone, uraemia, hypothyroidism, obstructive jaundice, raised intracranial pressure, glaucoma and drugs such as beta blockers and digoxin. Sinus bradycardia may be asymptomatic but in the presence of hypotension, heart failure or syncope, treatment is required.

Sinus tachycardia

Sinus tachycardia is due to the SA node discharging at a rate of 100/min or faster. This can be a physiological response to exercise or emotion. If the sinus tachycardia persists at rest, it can be due to a wide variety of disorders, such as anaemia, fever, thyrotoxicosis, infection, cardiac failure or pregnancy. Management should be directed towards diagnosing and treating the underlying condition. Sinus tachycardia should be distinguished from paroxysmal tachycardia, which starts and ends abruptly.

Sinus arrhythmia

The rate of the sinus node discharge alternates with periods of rapid rates and periods of slow rates. P waves are seen on the ECG and this rhythm is most commonly seen in children.

Sick sinus syndrome

This syndrome is characterized by inadequate function of the SA node, the AV nodes and its appendages. The sick sinus syndrome has many causes, including idiopathic fibrosis, ischaemic heart disease, cardiomyopathies and myocarditis. Due to impairment of the impulse conduction, sinus bradycardia, sinus arrest, sinoatrial block, atrial

tachycardias and extra systoles may occur. Sick sinus syndrome can occur in patients at any age but is most common in the elderly. It may present with dizziness, syncope or palpitation. The following abnormal rhythms may occur due to sick sinus syndrome. The abnormal rhythms are usually intermittent, sinus rhythm being present for the rest of the time.

1. Sinus bradycardia, which may cause lethargy or syncope, depending on its severity.
2. Sinus arrest. Sinus node activity ceases and thus the atria are not activated. No P waves are seen on the ECG. When the SA node fails, other pacemakers generate an escape rhythm.
3. Sinoatrial block. Impulses are blocked from leaving the sinoatrial node and thus fail to activate the atria.
4. Atrial tachycardias. Paroxysmal atrial fibrillation and atrial flutter may occur in patients with the sick sinus syndrome.
5. Atrial extrasystoles. These may be observed in healthy people but are mainly seen in patients with organic heart disease. They are often seen in the sick sinus syndrome and the ECG shows premature P waves, followed by a QRS complex and then a long pause.

Paroxysmal supraventricular tachycardia

This arrhythmia is due to the presence of an accessory electrical pathway between the atria and the ventricles. This allows the repeated circulation of an impulse between the atria and ventricles. The ECG shows a regular and usually narrow complex tachycardia. Normal P waves are not seen. The QRS complex rate is usually between 130 and 250/min.

Atrial flutter

In this arrhythmia, the atria discharge at a rate between 240 and 400 beats/min. The AV node usually blocks some of the atrial impulses: if the atrial rate is 300/min and the AV node blocks 50% of the impulses, then the ventricular rate is 150 beats/min. The ECG shows two P waves per QRS complex; this is called 2 : 1 block. In atrial flutter, the degree of block is variable.

Atrial fibrillation

In atrial fibrillation, the atria discharge at a rate of between 350 and 600/min. The AV node is unable to conduct all these electrical impulses to the ventricles, which contract at a slower rate than the atrial rate. The ventricles are excited in an irregular fashion, which results in an irregularly irregular pulse. The ECG does not show any P waves and the QRS complexes are completely irregular. Atrial fibrillation is a common arrhythmia and may be idiopathic, secondary to ischaemic heart disease, thyrotoxicosis, rheumatic fever, sick sinus syndrome, cardiomyopathy, myocarditis, pericarditis, congenital heart disease or pulmonary embolus.

6.2.3 Ventricular arrhythmias

Ventricular tachycardia

Ventricular tachycardia is defined as a series of three or more consecutive ventricular ectopic beats. The ECG shows a broad complex, regular tachycardia at a rate of 140–180/min. Ventricular tachycardia may have profound haemodynamic effects, leading to hypotension, loss of consciousness or heart failure. Although ventricular tachycardia can cause these serious symptoms and signs, it does not always do so.

Ventricular fibrillation

Ventricular fibrillation occurs most commonly following a myocardial infarction. Ventricular myocardial fibres propagate impulses in a totally disorganized fashion. The ECG shows irregular complexes in shape, size and rhythm. As the electrical activity of the ventricles is totally unco-ordinated in VF, there is no cardiac output, within a few seconds of the onset of VF, loss of consciousness and circulatory collapse occur.

Heart block

Heart block occurs in various diseases which causes the propagation of the electrical impulses to be slowed down or interrupted.

Atrioventricular block is characterized by slow or interrupted transmission of the atrial electrical activity to the ventricles as a result of abnormal conduction through the AV node.

First-degree AV block
The conduction of the atrial impulse through the AV node is delayed. The ECG shows a prolonged PR interval.

Second-degree AV block
The conduction of atrial impulses to the ventricles intermittently fails.

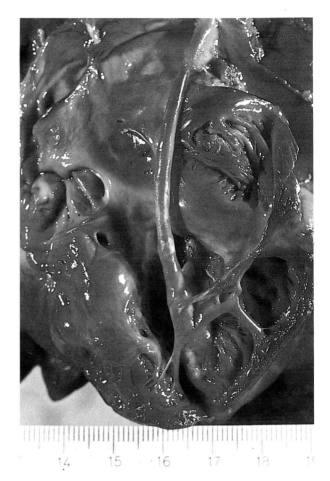

Fig. 6.7 Pacemaker probe in typical position.

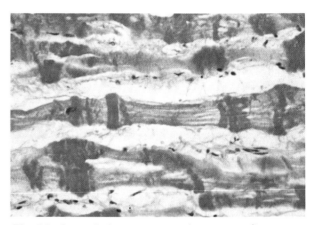

Fig. 6.8 Coagulation necroses of myocytes after defibrillation.

Mobitz Type I
In this type of second-degree block, the PR interval becomes progressively longer and eventually the atrial impulse fails to be conducted. After the dropped beat, the cycle repeats itself.

Mobitz Type II
In this type of second-degree AV block, the atrial

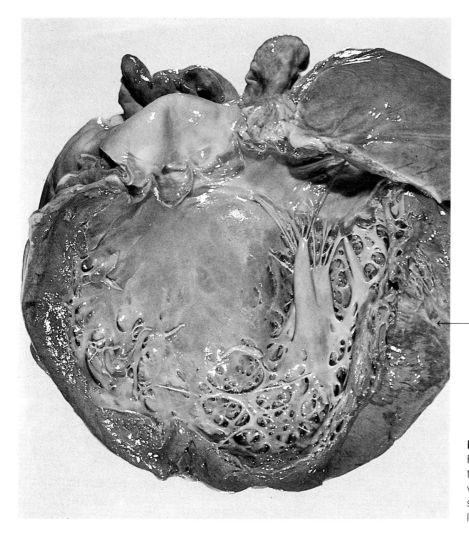

Fig. 6.9 Myocardial infarct.
Fresh myocardial necrosis in the posterior wall of the left ventricle (arrow). Balloon-shaped dilatation of ventricle lumen.

impulses which are conducted have a normal and constant PR interval. Some P waves, however, are not conducted through the AV node. The ratio of conducted to non-conducted beats may vary but usually there are two P waves per QRS complex.

Third-degree AV block
No atrial impulses pass through the AV node. The ventricles are stimulated by a slow escape rhythm usually from a pacemaker within the Bundle of His. There is no relationship between the P waves and the QRS complexes on the ECG.

Intraventricular block
The Bundle of His divides into two branches, the right and left bundle branches, which transmit the electrical impulses to the ventricular myocardium. If damage to either of these bundles occurs, an intraventricular conduction defect may result. Depending on which bundle is damaged, right or left bundle branch block ensues and this is diagnosed electrocardiographically.

Ventricular pre-excitation

The Wolff-Parkinson-White syndrome is caused by an accessory pathway between the atria and the ventricles. The accessory pathway does not delay the conduction of the impulse from the atria to the ventricles. The atrial impulses will reach the ventricles more quickly via the accessory pathway than via the normal route through the AV node. The accessory pathway predisposes to arrhythmias; atrial fibrillation and paroxysmal supraventricular tachycardia are the most commonly seen arrhythmias. The ECG of a patient with WPW syndrome shows a short PR interval, wide QRS complex with a delta wave, a slurred stroke on the upstroke of the R wave.

6.2.4   Pacemaker

A pacemaker consists of an impulse generator and a pacemaker wire with an electrode (Fig. 6.7). The tip of the electrode is usually positioned at the right ventricular apex. An electrical impulse can be conducted from the generator via the pacemaker wire to the ventricular myocardium and stimulate myocardial contraction. There are two types of pacemaker: temporary and permanent pacemakers. Temporary pacemakers are usually inserted following an anterior myocardial infarction, which has caused either third-degree AV block, second-degree AV block or bifascicular block. Temporary pacemakers are also inserted following an inferior myocardial infarction with second- or third-degree AV block, which causes hypotension, heart failure or syncope. Following a myocardial infarction, the heart block usually resolves within a couple of days and the temporary pacemaker can be removed. However, occasionally patients do require a permanent pacing post myocardial infarction. The indications for insertion of a permanent pacemaker include third-degree AV block with Stokes-Adams attacks, type II second-degree AV block, sick sinus syndrome and symptomatic patients with chronic bundle branch block.

6.2.5   Cardiac massage

Cardiac massage is required whenever the patient sustains a cardiac arrest. This means that there is sudden interruption of cardiac output, which may be reversible with appropriate treatment. Cardiac massage is a method of trying to maintain the circulation until appropriate treatment can be given to the patient to restore the circulation. To perform cardiac massage, the patient should be positioned to lie flat on his back, preferably on a hard surface. The hands should be positioned on the sternum just above the xiphisternum. The heel of one hand should be placed in the correct position on the sternum and the other hand placed on top of the first hand. The arms should be kept straight vertically above the hands and pressure applied to move the sternum 4cm downwards. The pressure should then be released. The rate of compression is 80/min. Possible complications of cardiac massage include

rib fractures, flail chest, myocardial haematomas and organ rupture.

6.2.6   Defibrillation

Defibrillation is the delivery of a large electrical shock to the heart muscle through the chest wall and is used to terminate ventricular fibrillatory cardiac arrest. The electrical shock causes depolarization of the myocardial cells, and if enough cells are depolarized, normal electrical activity may be restored. The electrical current itself may cause myocyte necrosis (Fig. 6.8).

6.2.7   DC cardioversion

DC cardioversion is the delivery of a large electrical shock to the heart muscle through the chest wall but differs from defibrillation in that the electrical shock is delivered at a particular point in the cardiac cycle. A synchronizing mechanism only allows the shock to be delivered when the R over S wave is detected by the machine. If the shock was delivered and coincided with the T wave, a VF arrest could occur. Defibrillation does not synchronize with any part of the electrical cycle. Cardioversion is used in the treatment of VT, atrial fibrillation and atrial flutter.

6.3   MYOCARDIAL INFARCTION (Fig. 6.9)

Ischaemic heart disease is the most common cause of death in industrialized nations. The average age for a first myocardial infarction in men is 60 years and five years later in women.

6.3.1   Pathogenesis

The onset of a myocardial infarction is usually triggered by the rupture of an athero-sclerotic plaque within a coronary artery. This induces thrombus formation and spasm of the coronary artery. The combination of the ruptured plaque, thrombus formation and vessel spasm may occlude the coronary artery, inducing myocardial ischaemia. The ischaemic myocardium does not die immediately following coronary artery occlusion but the metabolic function of the ischaemic tissue gradually deteriorates and the damage becomes irreversible (necrosis) after approximately six hours of ischaemia. Occasionally, myocardial infarction may occur as a result of an embolus lodging in a

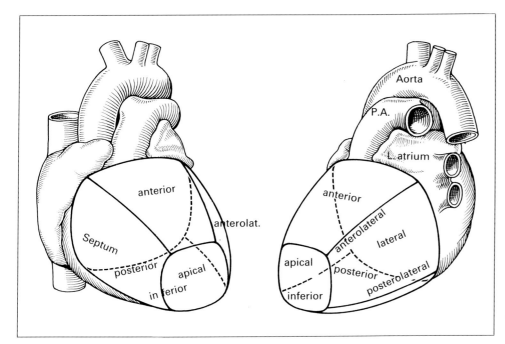

Fig. 6.10 Site and extent of myocardial infarcts.

normal coronary artery and occluding it. Embolism may occur from mitral stenosis or subacute bacterial endocarditis. Myocardial infarctions may also occasionally occur due to reduced coronary blood flow secondary to such disorders as systolic hypotension, constrictive pericarditis or pericardial tamponade, which may all severely impair the blood flow through the coronary artery and induce myocardial ischaemia. Myocardial infarction most commonly occurs as a result of coronary artery disease but myocardial infarctions may occur in patients with normal coronary arteries if an embolus occludes the coronary artery or some other process severely impairs myocardial perfusion, such as severe systolic hypertension, etc. Myocardial infarctions in younger patients are those occurring before the age of 40 in men and 50 in women. Risk factors which predispose to myocardial infarction include cigarette smoking, hypertension, hypercholesterolaemia, diabetes, positive family history of ischaemic heart disease and obesity.

6.3.2 Sudden cardiac death

Sudden cardiac death is an unexpected cardiac death occurring without symptoms or with symptoms of less than an hour's duration. The most common cause of sudden cardiac death is ischaemic heart disease: either myocardial ischaemia or infarction precipitates VF. Sudden cardiac death

usually occurs outside hospital and is a common cause of mortality in 20–60-year-old patients. Sudden cardiac death may also be caused by myocarditis, cardiomyopathy, hypertensive cardiac hypertrophy, acute or chronic valve defects and acute or chronic cor pulmonale.

6.3.3 Site of myocardial infarction

Myocardial infarct size and site (Fig. 6.10) are important factors in determining the outcome of the patient, post myocardial infarction. Anterior myocardial infarcts tend to be larger and are associated with more significant impairment of left ventricular function and carry a higher mortality than inferior myocardial infarcts. Anterior and inferior infarcts are the most common sites for a myocardial infarction. The terms anterior, inferior, septal, lateral and posterior are used to describe the site of a myocardial infarction and refer to myocardial infarctions involving the left ventricle. Right ventricular infarctions are rare and usually occur in conjunction with left ventricular posterior infarctions.

A transmural infarction affects all the layers of the ventricular wall. More than 90% of the immediate deaths from ischaemic heart disease are due to transmural infarctions.

A subendocardial infarction affects only the subendocardial part of the ventricular wall. Many

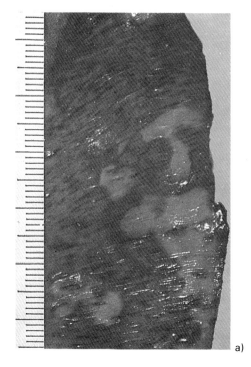

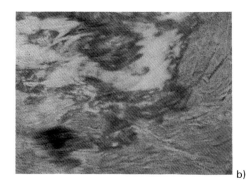

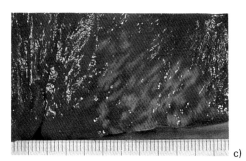

Fig. 6.11 Myocardial infarct.
a) Clay-coloured incision surface of myocardium with a fresh infarct.
b) Myocardial infarct undergoing organization, with haemorrhagic margin.
c) Old myocardial infarct scar.

clinical studies have shown that subendocardial myocardial infarctions have a similar mortality to transmural myocardial infarctions.

Large infarctions

Myocardial necrosis greater than 2.5cm in diameter is called a macro infarct. Micro infarcts are less than 2.5cm in diameter.

Myocytolysis

This is a pathological term used to describe the result of ischaemic injury (Fig. 6.11a). The myocytes are damaged but survive for a time. Histologically, the cell membrane remains intact but the intracellular structures degenerate and the cell ultimately dies (Figs 6.11b,c).

A paradoxical infarct: the localization of the myocardial necrosis does not correspond with the vascular pattern. This type of infarct occurs after vascular occlusion in chronic coronary disease where the formation of collateral vessels has led to the supply of areas of myocardium with other arterial branches.

6.3.4 Pathology of myocardial infarction

Macroscopic features

The macroscopic pathological changes are not visible until eight hours after the myocardial infarction. Initially, an area of pale, soft myocardium is detected. If the infarct has been large, fibrinous pericarditis may be found. A week after the myocardial infarct, an area of granulation tissue, rich in capillaries, is found surrounding the infarcted area. Organization of the necrotic tissue occurs and eventually a fibrous scar, composed of collagen (Fig. 6.12), is formed.

Histology

Following a myocardial infarction, myocardial fibre oedema develops over 30–60 min. After two hours the sarcoplasma becomes homogenous and then clumps together with small hyperchromatic nuclei. The necrosis is fully evident after 4–6h with intensive sarcoplasmic eosinophilia, degeneration of the muscle fibres (sarcolysis); the sarcolemma appears

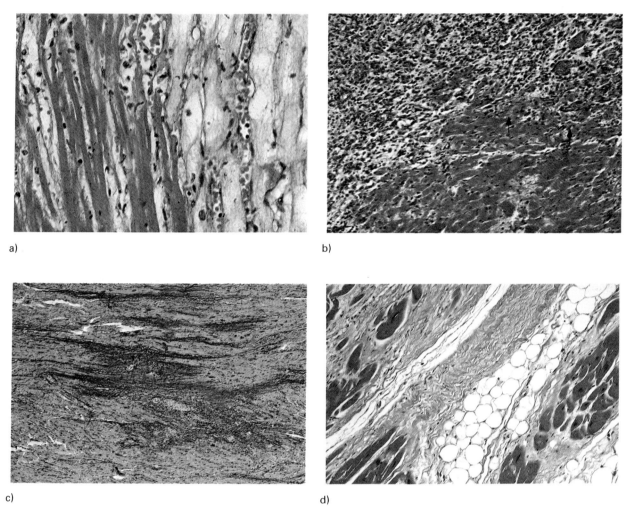

Fig. 6.12 a) Myocytolysis. b) Myocardial infarct with granulation tissue (arrow = infarct residue). c) Old myocardial scar, van-Gieson red. d) Fat cell growth in an old myocardial scar. HE staining.

empty with loss of the cross-striations and nuclear outlines. Capillaries filled with blood invade the margins of the necrosis, followed by granulocytes. This phase lasts 18–24h.

Myocardial infarction undergoing organization

Over a period of two to three weeks, the necrotic tissue is broken down and replaced by granulation tissue. Necrotic remains can be detected in the centre, surrounded by granulation tissue containing many capillaries. There are also histiocytes which may store pigments such as haemosiderin and lipofuscin. The newly formed collagen fibres are still sparse in this phase. After some months, a scar with an irregular outline, poor in cells and capillaries but rich in fibres, can be seen as a replacement for the necrotic myocardium. The newly formed van Gieson red collagen fibres are at first delicate but later become thick and hyalinized. The surrounding myocytes are hypertrophied (large, barrel-shaped nuclei).

6.3.5 Clinical features of myocardial infarction

In more than 60% of patients with myocardial infarction, there is sudden onset of severe, prolonged, restrosternal chest pain, which may radiate to the arms, neck, or jaw and is unrelieved by rest or nitroglycerin. The patient may also describe dyspnoea, acute anxiety, sweating, palpitations, dizziness and especially with inferior or posterior myocardial infarctions, nausea and vomiting. The patient usually describes the chest pain as a tightness or heaviness. In up to 20% of cases, the myocardial infarct may pass unnoticed, i.e. a silent myocardial infarct, and this usually occurs in elder-

Stage		ECG trace	Features
normal			1. Small Q 2. High R 3. ST isoelectric 4. T upright
fresh infarct (acute stage)	Stage 1		1. Marked ST elevation 2. T positive 3. Small R 4. Q still small
	Intermediate stage		1. Slight ST elevation 2. T wave inverted 3. Large Q 4. Small R
old infarct (chronic stage)	Stage 2		1. T wave inverted 2. Large Q 3. R still small 4. No ST elevation
	Stage 3		1. Q still pathological 2. T now positive 3. Normal R 4. No ST elevation

Fig. 6.13 ECG with myocardial infarct.

ly or diabetic patients. The patient has no specific symptoms or arrhythmias. Another group of patients with myocardial infarcts will present with atypical symptoms. Thus the presentation of a myocardial infarct can be with typical symptoms, atypical symptoms or silent.

Physical examination

The findings on physical examination are influenced by the site and size of the myocardial infarct and also if the patient has a past medical history of myocardial infarction. The most common physical findings are those of left ventricular failure, such as triple rhythm, pulmonary crepitations, tachycardia or hypotension. Many patients, following a myocardial infarct, will have no abnormal physical findings if the infarct is small and they have remained in sinus rhythm, with reasonable ventricular function.

Diagnosis of myocardial infarction

ECG
The ECG gives decisive evidence for the presence of

a myocardial infarct, which reveals a typical sequence of ECG changes with time. The ECG also gives an indication as to the site of myocardial infarction.

Transmural myocardial infarction
Acute stage In the acute stage, the ECG shows ST elevation. This occurs within a few hours of the onset of the myocardial infarct.

Fully evolved stage This usually occurs within the first 24h. Pathological Q waves are seen with ST elevation and T wave inversion.

Resolution phase Pathological Q waves are seen. The ST segments and T waves have usually returned to normal but changes can persist for a long time following the infarct.

Subendocardial myocardial infarction
The ECG shows symmetrical T wave inversion. The ECG leads which manifest the ECG changes indicate the site of the myocardial infarction.

Anterior myocardial infarction
Anterior myocardial infarctions are sub-divided into:

1. Extensive anterior myocardial infarctions in which the ECG changes are seen in I, aVL and standard leads V1–V6.
2. Anteroseptal myocardial infarction. The ECG changes are seen in V1–V4.
3. Anterolateral myocardial infarction. The ECG changes are seen in V4–V6, I, and aVL.
4. Inferior myocardial infarction. The ECG changes are seen in leads II, III and aVF.

Laboratory parameters
Further evidence to help in the diagnosis of myocardial infarction is provided by a characteristic pattern of cardiac enzyme changes in the blood. The necrotic myocardium releases intracellular enzymes into the blood and these can be measured.

CPK (creatinine phosphokinase; MB isoenzyme) A rise in this isoenzyme is specific for heart muscle necrosis. The blood levels rise within a few hours of the myocardial infarction and fall within 72h.

AST (aspartate transaminase) This enzyme rises in the blood 12–24h following a myocardial infarction and returns to normal levels usually within five days. Raised AST levels are also found in liver disease, pulmonary emboli or muscle injury, so it is not as specific an enzyme as CKMB for myocardial damage.

LDH (lactate dehydrogenase) This enzyme is not cardiac specific. The levels following a myocardial infarct rise slowly and remain elevated for approximately ten days. This enzyme can be raised in haematological diseases, renal disease, liver disease or muscle disease.

Other laboratory investigations
Non-specific findings following myocardial infarction include a raised ESR or a raised white cell count. The blood glucose can be raised transiently following a myocardial infarction.

The diagnosis of a myocardial infarction is usually based on the clinical history, typical sequential ECG changes and a characteristic rise and fall in cardiac enzymes. The vast majority of myocardial infarctions are diagnosed on these criteria. However, occasionally other investigations are required.

Imaging procedures
The imaging procedures used to aid in the diag-

nosis of a myocardial infarction are myocardial scintigraphy and echocardiography.

Myocardial scintigraphy The radio-nuclear substances Indium-III labelled antimyosin and technetium-99m labelled pyrophosphate both accumulate in acutely infarcted myocardium. Either of these substances can be used to image the heart of a patient who has sustained a possible myocardial infarction, to try to confirm or refute the diagnosis. These techniques are not used commonly. An example of a clinical situation when these tests would be used would be for patients with long-standing left bundle branch block on their ECG and the results of the cardiac enzymes were equivocal following an episode of chest pain. The ECG in this type of patient cannot be interpreted to confirm or exclude a myocardial infarction and the cardiac enzyme results are unhelpful.

Echocardiography The echocardiogram can demonstrate segmental ventricular wall motion abnormalities suggestive of myocardial infarction but the echo cannot give evidence of when the wall motion abnormality was sustained.

Prognosis

The prognosis of patients following myocardial infarction is influenced by many factors but the major determinant of survival is the amount of myocardium that has been infarcted. A poor prognosis is indicated by any of the following: an anterior myocardial infarction, heart failure, hypotension, recurrent chest pain post myocardial infarction, arrhythmias and/or conduction abnormalities on the ECG. If a patient is diabetic or has had a previous myocardial infarction, or is over 65, there is an increased mortality.

Ventricular fibrillation

Ventricular fibrillation is the most common cause of death in the first few hours following a myocardial infarction. It is estimated that approximately 25% of all patients with a myocardial infarction die before reaching hospital. Of all the myocardial infarction patients who reach hospital alive, approximately 80% are discharged alive. Of the patients discharged, approximately 10% will die in the next year. The overall survival for patients post myocardial infarction at one year is approximately 55%.

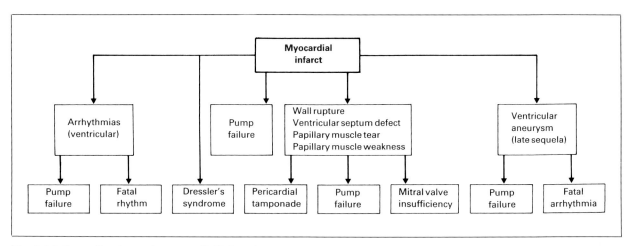

Fig. 6.14 Complications of myocardial infarction.

Treatment of cardiac arrhythmias

Arrhythmia	Treatment
Ventricular fibrillation (VF)	Defibrillation.
Ventricular tachycardia (VT)	DC cardioversion. Class I anti-arrhythmic drugs.
Ventricular premature beats (VPBs)	Treatment is required if there are R on T ectopics, if the VPBs are multi-focal in origin or if there are salvoes of VPBs. Treatment is a Class I anti-arrhythmic drug.
Sinus tachycardia	Treatment of the underlying cause, e.g. congestive heart failure, infection.
Atrial fibrillation	Cardioversion is used if the patient is haemodynamically compromised. If the patient is stable, drug therapy, such as beta blockers, digoxin or amiodarone can be given.
Atrial flutter	Cardioversion can be used if the patient is haemodynamically compromised and is the best form of treatment for atrial flutter. However, digoxin, beta blockers and amiodarone can also be used in the treatment of this arrhythmia.
Sinus bradycardia	No treatment is required if the patient is not haemodynamically compromised and is asymptomatic. If, however, a patient is haemodynamically compromised, intravenous atropine should be given and, if necessary, a temporary pacemaker inserted if the arrhythmia is resistant to atropine.
1st-degree heart block	If the patient is haemodynamically compromised atropine should be given. A temporary pacemaker may be required if the arrhythmia is resistant to atropine or bifascicular block is present on the ECG.
2nd-degree heart block	If a patient is haemodynamically compromised, has an anterior myocardial infarction or has associated right bundle branch block/left bundle branch block or bifascicular block, a temporary pacemaker is required.
3rd-degree heart block	If a patient is haemodynamically compromised or has had an anterior myocardial infarction or has associated right bundle branch block/left bundle branch block or bifascicular block on the ECG, a temporary pacemaker is required.

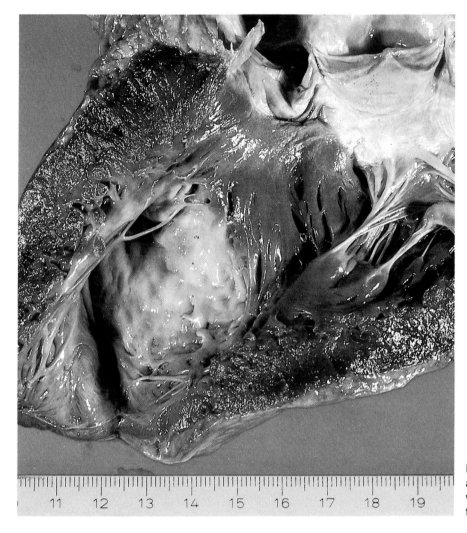

Fig. 6.15 Long-standing cardiac aneurysm in the septal area with concomitant endocardial thickening.

6.3.6 Complications of myocardial infarctions

Cardiac arrhythmias

These are the most common complications of myocardial infarction. They range from life-threatening VF arrest to a mild bradycardia or tachycardia which requires no treatment. For details of treatment, see p. 66.

Acute left heart failure

Acute left heart failure is an emergency and is seen in 25% of patients with acute myocardial infarction. Precipitating causes of left heart failure, in addition to the myocardial infarction, should be sought and treated, e.g. 3rd degree heart block would require a temporary pacemaker. The patient should be treated, whilst kept sitting up, with oxygen, in-travenous morphine and intravenous diuretics. If the blood pressure is satisfactory and further treatment is required, intravenous nitrates can be given.

Cardiogenic shock

Post myocardial infarction, patients who develop cardiogenic shock have a very high mortality of at least 80%. It usually occurs in patients who have severe underlying coronary artery disease, who have had large myocardial infarctions resulting in severe left ventricular dysfunction. The clinical features of cardiogenic shock are hypotension, oliguria, cool, pale, moist skin and impaired cerebration.

A Swan-Ganz catheter should be inserted to allow accurate haemodynamic monitoring. Diuretics may be used to lower the left ventricular filling pressure. The contractility of the myocardium may be improved with inotropes such as dobutamine or

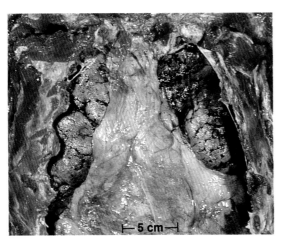

Fig. 6.16 Pericardial tamponade.

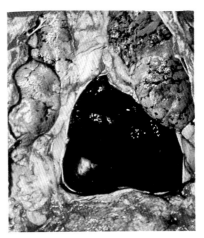

Fig. 6.17 Pericardial cavity filled with a blood clot.

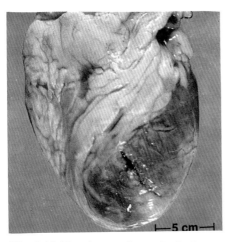

Fig. 6.18 Tear in anterior wall of left ventricle after myocardial infarct.

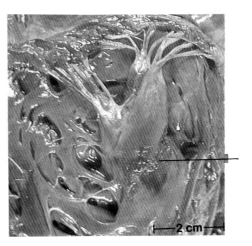

Fig. 6.19 Tear of a mitral papillary muscle in myocardial infarct.

dopamine. If the systolic blood pressure can be maintained at at least 90mmHg, vasodilator therapy, such as intravenous nitrates, may be introduced in an attempt to reduce the afterload. Cardiogenic shock post myocardial infarction is usually due to extensive myocardial necrosis but can occur due to a post infarction VSD or mitral valve regurgitation. These conditions should be sought as they can be treated surgically.

Dressler's syndrome

This syndrome consists of a prolonged intermittent fever, pericarditis, pleural effusions and a high ESR. It is believed to be autoimmune in origin and occurs in approximately 5% of post myocardial infarction patients, usually one to four weeks following their myocardial infarction. The treatment is initially non-steroidal anti-inflammatory drugs and, if indicated, steroids.

Left ventricular aneurysm

This can occur in up to 10% of all myocardial infarction patients (Fig. 6.15). The most common presentation is persistent ST elevation on the ECG. This diagnosis can be confirmed by echocardiography, MUGA scan or a left ventriculogram. The complications which may occur due to the left ventricular aneurysm include arterial emboli, arrhythmias, heart failure and, rarely, rupture of the myocardial wall.

Thrombo-embolic complications

These can occur in 10–40% of patients post myocardial infarction. The formation of systemic emboli is favoured by the presence of increasing patient age, congestive heart failure, anterior myocardial infarction, left ventricular aneurysm or left ventricular

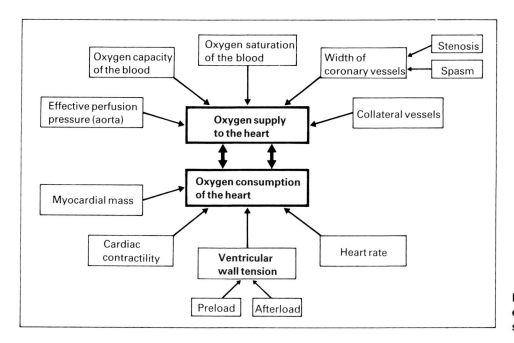

Fig. 6.20 Equilibrium of cardiac oxygen supply and demand.

hypertrophy. Arterial embolization usually occurs one to three weeks post myocardial infarction.

Pulmonary emboli

Deep venous thrombosis is relatively common post myocardial infarction, occurring in 10–35% of patients. Risk factors for the development of a deep venous thrombosis include increased patient age, congestive heart failure, diuretics, cardiogenic shock, obesity, previous pulmonary embolism or prolonged bed rest. In order to prevent deep venous thrombosis formation, patients are mobilized early post myocardial infarction and if any of the above risk factors are present, prophylactic heparin should be considered.

Cardiac tamponade

Rupture of the myocardium is a common cause of death following a large myocardial infarction.

Acquired ventricular septal defect

If the interventricular septum is damaged by the myocardial infarction, it may perforate, resulting in a ventricular septal defect. This causes a rapid deterioration in the patient's haemodynamic status. Examination reveals a new systolic murmur loudest at the left sternal edge. The diagnosis may be confirmed using a Swan-Ganz catheter to detect a step-up in the oxygen saturation in the right ventricular blood due to the presence of the shunt.

Surgery can be performed to close the defect but there is a high mortality from this complication of myocardial infarction.

Mitral regurgitation

Mitral regurgitation may result from papillary muscle damage post myocardial infarction. The severity of the mitral regurgitation depends on the severity of the papillary muscle dysfunction. Papillary muscle dysfunction may result in transient mitral regurgitation with no significant haemodynamic consequences and this has a good prognosis. However, if the muscle actually ruptures, severe mitral regurgitation causes acute pulmonary oedema. The systolic murmur of a ventricular septal defect may be difficult to differentiate from the murmur of mitral regurgitation and a Swan-Ganz catheter may help in the diagnosis. A ventricular septal defect causes a left to right shunt with step-up in oxygen saturation in the right ventricular blood. In mitral regurgitation, there is no shunt and thus no step-up in the right ventricular oxygen saturation. Severe mitral regurgitation can be treated surgically but has a high mortality. Mild mitral regurgitation does not require surgical treatment and is often transient.

Pericarditis

This is a relatively common complication of myocardial infarction. The patient usually complains of a sharp pleuritic chest pain, which is relieved with

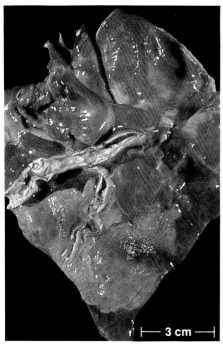

Fig. 6.21 Coronary sclerosis of the elastic type without lumen narrowing.

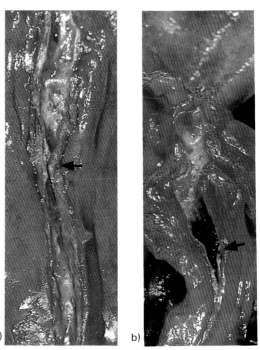

Fig. 6.22 a) coronary sclerosis with waist-like constriction of lumen; b) coronary thrombosis.

sitting forward. A friction rub may be heard on auscultation. Pericarditis is treated with non-steroidal anti-inflammatory drugs and usually settles within a few days.

Cardiac arrest

Cardiac arrest is the cessation of an effective cardiac output as a result of a sudden circulatory or respiratory catastrophe. The three arrhythmias which commonly cause cardiac arrest post myocardial infarction are: ventricular fibrillation, asystole and electro-mechanical dissociation. Of these three arrhythmias, ventricular fibrillation has the best prognosis and the treatment of this arrhythmia has already been discussed.

Asystole

Asystole is characterized by ventricular standstill due to the suppression of the natural pacemakers in the heart. The ECG shows no ventricular activity and cardio-pulmonary resuscitation should be commenced immediately. Asystole is treated with adrenaline intravenously, atropine intravenously and if this is unsuccessful, temporary pacing should be considered.

Electromechanical dissociation

This is due to myocardial pump failure despite normal electrical activity within the heart. The ECG shows normal cardiac rhythm but the patient has no cardiac output. Electromechanical dissociation can be caused by myocardial infarction but can also be caused by pulmonary embolus, tension pneumothorax, cardiac tamponade, myocardial rupture or severe blood loss. The management of electromechanical dissociation involves identifying any precipitating cause and the treatment of the precipitating cause. If electromechanical dissociation has occurred following myocardial infarction, it is treated with adrenaline intravenously and then calcium chloride intravenously should be considered. Electromechanical dissociation has a poor prognosis.

In addition to the physical complications of myocardial infarction, there can be psychological and social complications. Some patients may lose their jobs following a myocardial infarction and may experience either anxiety or depression.

6.4 CORONARY HEART DISEASE (CHD)

Coronary heart disease is a common condition in the industrialized countries and is due to atherosclerotic thickening of the coronary arteries. The term CHD, when used clinically, refers to the spectrum of disease covered by angina, myocardial infarction and sudden cardiac death.

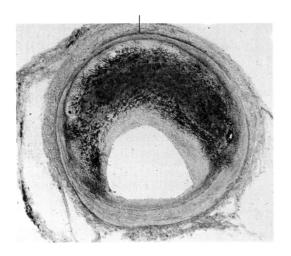

Fig. 6.23 Coronary sclerosis. Arrow = media. Sudan staining.

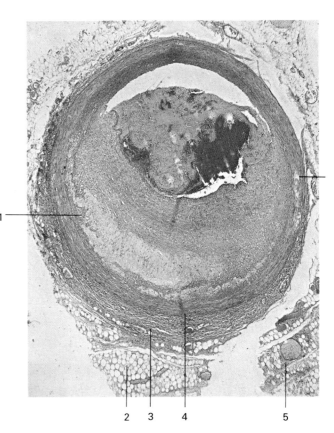

Fig. 6.24 Coronary sclerosis with constriction of lumen. 1: intima with atheroma. 2: adventitia. 3: media. 4: elastica interna. 5: nerve. HE staining.

Risk factors for CHD

Cigarette smoking
Male sex
Increasing age
Hyperlipidaemia
Hypertension
Family history of CHD
Obesity
Diabetes
Gout

Hyperlipidaemia

The myocardial infarction rate increases linearly with the blood cholesterol level. Hypercholesterolaemia may have a genetic basis or be due to a poor diet with a high proportion of saturated fat and lack of physical activity.

Hypertension

Hypertension increases mortality and facilitates the progression of atherosclerosis.

6.4.1 Pathophysiology of CHD

Angina pectoris is caused by an imbalance between myocardial oxygen supply and demand, which results in myocardial oxygen deficiency. This is expressed via vagal and sympathetic nerve fibres as pain or discomfort, which is usually retrosternal in site but can radiate to the arms, back or throat.

Reduced myocardial oxygen supply can be due to either a stenosis of a coronary artery impairing blood flow to the myocardium, or reduced oxygen carried in the blood, e.g. due to anaemia or pulmonary disease. Conditions which increase myocardial oxygen demand are physical effort, anger, heavy meals or exposure to cold.

6.4.2 Pathology of CHD

Athero-sclerosis consists of plaques of intimal thickening of artery walls due to the accumulation of lipid and fibrous tissue.

Macroscopic appearances

The coronary artery has yellow/white plaques in its intima which reduce the cross-sectional area of the lumen (Figs 6.21–6.24). Rupture of a plaque exposes underlying collagen which promotes thrombosis which may occlude the artery causing a myocardial infarction.

71

Histology

The main histological feature of an atherosclerotic plaque is the accumulation of lipid within the intima with overlying fibrous tissue. Sudan staining colours of lipid intimal deposits orange-red. Other features which may be seen include calcification, vessel media atrophy and macrophages laden with lipid. With HE staining, pale areas can be seen within the thickened intima corresponding to extracted lipid and in the vessel wall there are numerous calcifications coloured blue. If thrombosis occurs, the lumen is occluded by a thrombus composed of platelets and fibrin. The elastica interna may demonstrate evidence of splitting with the formation of new elastic fibres.

6.4.3 Clinical features of CHD

The major forms of CHD include angina pectoris, myocardial infarction and sudden cardiac death.

Angina pectoris

Angina pectoris is an acute transient myocardial insufficiency of oxygen which is usually precipitated by exertion or emotion. The pain can be relieved by rest or nitroglycerin and usually lasts less than five minutes.

Unstable angina

This form of angina is manifested by a sudden increase in the frequency of onset of anginal attacks and they occur at rest or in minimal exertion. Unstable angina may progress to myocardial infarction.

Prinzmetal's angina

The pain of Prinzmetal's angina is typical of classic angina except that the pain occurs at rest, often in a predictable pattern. If an ECG is done during an episode of chest pain, ST elevation is seen. The pain is relieved with nitroglycerin but usually after 20–30min. This condition is due to spasm of the coronary artery which may, or may not, have atherosclerosis.

Diagnosis of angina

The case history is of great importance in diagnosing angina. If typical angina symptoms are described by the patient, then significant narrowing of the coronary artery is present in over 75% of men and about 60% of women. Physical examination may reveal signs of hypertension, hyperlipidaemia, anaemia or heart failure. There are no clinical signs of angina per se but there may be signs of predisposing factors or of the complications.

ECG

The resting ECG of a patient with angina usually reveals no abnormality, unless the patient has previously sustained a myocardial infarction. If the ECG is taken during an anginal episode, then ST elevation or depression is seen.

The exercise ECG

The exercise ECG is a non-invasive test which is used in the diagnosis of angina. Patients are exercised on a treadmill or bicycle according to a standard protocol, whilst having ECGs taken. The exercise induces angina which causes ST depression on the ECG. The exercise ECG can be used to confirm the diagnosis and also allows assessment of the patient's exercise capacity. The exercise ECG is positive in 40–80% of patients with CHD. The sensitivity of the test increases as the severity of the CHD increases, i.e. in mild CHD only 40% of patients will have positive tests but in severe CHD 80% will be positive. The test can also be falsely positive, i.e. a positive test but normal coronary arteries.

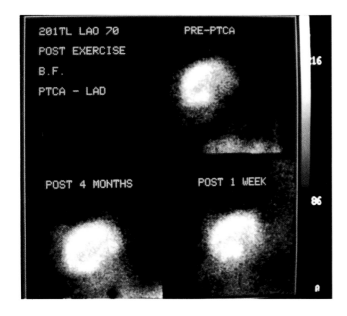

Fig. 6.25 Thallium scintigram in myocardial ischaemia.

Myocardial perfusion scanning

Thallium-201 is a radio-isotope which distributes itself in the myocardium after intravenous injection. If an area of myocardium is underperfused due to CHD, then less thallium will accumulate in that area. If myocardial ischaemia (Fig. 6.25) is induced, either by exercise or IV dipyridamole and then the radio-isotope is injected, the areas of ischaemic myocardium take up less thallium than the areas that are normally perfused. A second scan is performed four hours later without inducing myocardial ischaemia, using IV dipyridamole or exercise. If an area is ischaemic on the first scan but has normal perfusion on the second scan, then that area of myocardium is said to have reversible myocardial ischaemia. If, however, an area is underperfused on both scans, this is suggestive of a fixed perfusion defect probably due to previous myocardial infarction. The dipyridamole thallium study is a very useful non-invasive test in the diagnosis of patients who may have angina but are unable to perform exercise satisfactorily for an exercise test. The patient may have arthritis,

pulmonary disease, etc. and be unable to exercise sufficiently to induce myocardial ischaemia, as a result of their non-cardiac problems. The thallium scan is approximately 80% sensitive and the sensitivity increases with the severity of the CHD.

Laboratory tests

There is no laboratory test for the diagnosis of angina but patients who present with angina should have their blood glucose, cholesterol and haemoglobin checked.

Coronary angiography

This is an invasive investigation used to confirm the diagnosis and/or severity of CHD. It can also be used to assess left ventricular function. This investigation demonstrates the severity and extent of atherosclerotic lesions in the coronary arteries. Angiography is used to plan further treatment for patients with severe CHD, e.g. angioplasty or bypass surgery.

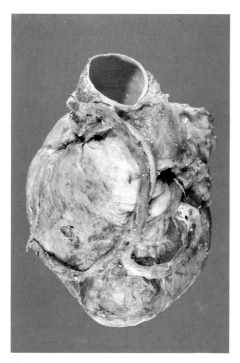

Fig. 6.26 Aorto-coronary bypass. Connection between aorta and peripheral sectors of both coronary arteries via bypass.

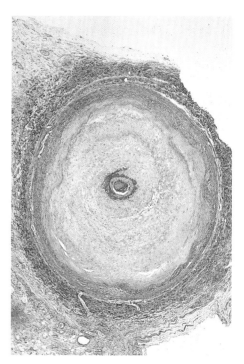

Fig. 6.27 Bypass with lumen stenosis due to concentric intima fibrosis. HE staining.

6.5 AORTO-CORONARY BYPASS

A piece of saphenous vein is inserted between the aorta and the post-stenotic part of the coronary artery. This acts as a bypass, allowing blood to flow beyond the narrowed segment of the coronary artery (Figs 6.26–6.27). The indications for bypass surgery include left main coronary artery disease, severe anginal symptoms despite optimal medical therapy, or angina and intolerance of medical therapy. The prerequisites for bypass surgery are lesions on the angiogram suitable for grafting and satisfactory LV function. The early mortality post operatively is less than 2% and depends on the pre-operative LV function and the experience of the surgical team. The symptoms of angina are relieved in 85% of patients one year after the operation, and at five years post operation approximately 70% will be pain-free. The pathological changes in the vein graft post operatively include concentric deposits of fibrin microthrombi along the venous intima and intimal proliferation may be observed one month post operatively. Progressively, the implanted veins may develop features of atherosclerosis. This may manifest as recurrence of angina post operatively, or acute myocardial infarction. The native arteries may also undergo atherosclerotic changes with time, so angina some years post operatively may be due to graft or native vessel atherosclerosis.

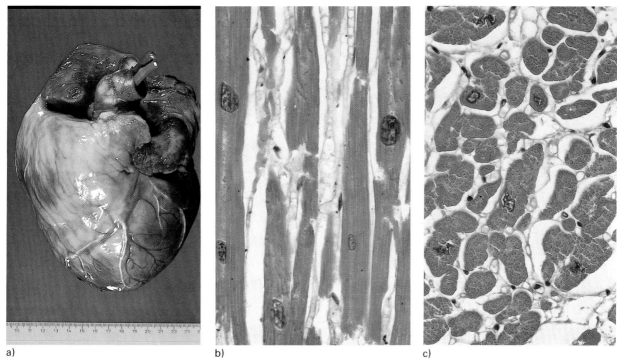

Fig. 6.28 Primary dilated cardiomyopathy. a) Greatly dilated heart with left hypertrophy. b) Thin muscle fibres with hyperchromatic, enlarged nuclei in longitudinal section. c) Enlarged and bizarre myocardial muscle nuclei in cross-section. HE staining.

6.6 CARDIOMYOPATHIES

Cardiomyopathies are disorders of cardiac muscle of unknown aetiology. They can be classified as follows:

1. Dilated (congestive) cardiomyopathy
2. Hypertrophic cardiomyopathy
3. Restrictive cardiomyopathy

6.6.1 Dilated cardiomyopathy

In this condition, the myocardium becomes dilated and contracts poorly (Fig. 6.28). The incidence is 7.3 cases per 100 000 head of population and men are affected 2–7 times more commonly than women. The peak age of onset is 40–59 years of age.

Pathology

The heart is dilated and flabby with patchy fibrosis. There may be mild hypertrophy of the ventricles. Histologically, there is hypertrophy of the muscle fibres which may vary markedly in size. The nuclei are bizarrely shaped. The interstitial tissue is fibrotic and there is no cellular infiltrate. Electron microscopy shows increased numbers of mitochondria.

Clinical features

The patients present with symptoms and signs of biventricular failure, although left ventricular failure may predominate. The diagnosis is based on exclusion of other specific causes of congestive heart failure. The prognosis is poor and the mortality rate is 34% within one year of diagnosis.

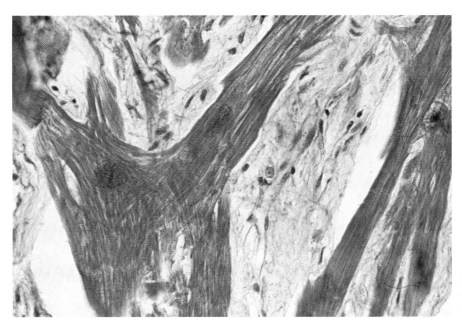

Fig. 6.29 Primary hypertrophic cardiomyopathy with bizarre myocytes. HE staining.

6.6.2 Hypertrophic cardiomyopathy

This is known by various synonyms such as hypertrophic obstructive cardiomyopathy (Fig. 6.29), idiopathic hypertrophic subvalvular aortic stenosis, or asymmetric septal hypertrophy.

Hypertrophic cardiomyopathy has the following characteristic findings:

1. Asymmetric hypertrophy of the septum with or without narrowing of the left ventricular outflow tract.
2. Systolic anterior movement of the anterior mitral cusp.

The histological features include myocyte hypertrophy with the muscle fibres arranged in bizarre, sometimes spiral patterns. Electron microscopy reveals myocyte hypertrophy with disturbances of the orientation and organization of the myocytes and myofibrils.

Clinical features

Hypertrophic cardiomyopathy may be an asymptomatic condition, or it can cause severe symptoms. It can be transmitted in an autosomal dominant fashion and affects the sexes equally. The abnormal myocardium in hypertrophic cardiomyopathy is stiff and this causes impairment of ventricular filling in diastole. Forms of hypertrophic cardiomyopathy with and without obstruction are distinguished. The presence of obstruction means that the asymmetric hypertrophied septum obstructs the left ventricular outflow tract. Thus, hypertrophic cardiomyopathy without obstruction will present with symptoms and signs due to left ventricular dysfunction. If obstruction is present, this will cause additional symptoms and signs. The clinical features of hypertrophic cardiomyopathy are varied. Patients may present with dyspnoea, angina, palpitations, syncope, dizziness or sudden death. Patients may also be asymptomatic and hypertrophic cardiomyopathy is found on routine examination or screening. The clinical signs include a jerky pulse, systolic murmur and distinctive apical beat. The ECG may be normal or show signs of left ventricular hypertrophy with ST and T wave changes, Q waves in the inferior and septal leads, ventricular ectopics and Wolff-Parkinson-White syndrome.

Echocardiography

The echocardiogram shows left ventricular hypertrophy especially of the septum, which has reduced motion. Systolic anterior movement of the mitral valve is seen, as is a small left ventricular cavity. The aortic valve is seen to close in mid systole and there is reduced diastolic closure rate of the mitral valve.

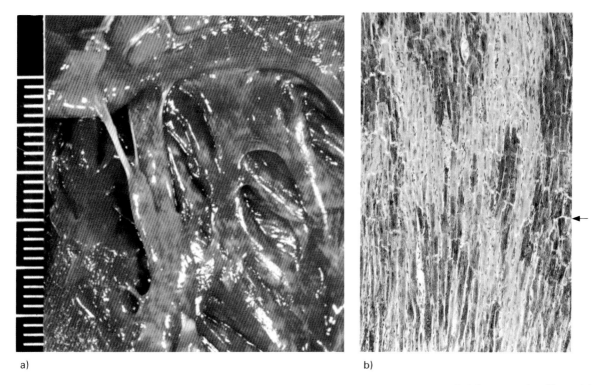

a)   b)

Fig. 6.30 a) Heart muscle with tiger stripes in oxygen deficiency. b) Fatty myocardial degeneration (tiger stripes). Sudan-haematoxylin staining.

Cardiac catheterization

This demonstrates raised systolic and end diastolic pressures. The outflow tract pressure gradient can be measured. Left ventriculography confirms the presence of a massively thickened septum, with left ventricular outflow obstruction. The left ventricular cavity has a normal shape. The coronary arteries usually have no evidence of athero-sclerosis.

The complications of hypertrophic cardiomyopathy are congestive heart failure, arrhythmias and sudden cardiac death.

Hypertrophic cardiomyopathy usually presents in younger adults and has an annual mortality rate of 2.5%. Treatment of this condition is mainly symptomatic, using beta blockers to improve dyspnoea, angina and palpitation. Ventricular arrhythmias are a common cause of death in hypertrophic cardiomyopathy, and all patients should have an exercise test and 24-h tape to try to detect possible arrhythmias. If arrhythmias are detected, the appropriate drug should be commenced and the exercise and 24-h tape repeated to see if the arrhythmia has been suppressed by the drug.

Amiodarone has been found to be a very useful drug in the treatment of arrhythmias in hypertrophic cardiomyopathy.

6.6.3 Restrictive cardiomyopathy

Restrictive cardiomyopathy is an uncommon disorder in which the systolic function of the ventricles is normal but the ventricular filling is impaired as a result of excessive ventricular rigidity during diastole. Restrictive cardiomyopathies include two pathological states which cannot always be differentiated.

6.6.4 Tropical endomyocardial fibrosis

Tropical endomyocardial fibrosis is largely restricted to the African continent. Endomyocardial scarring occurs, which can affect either or both ventricles, resulting in impairment of diastolic function.

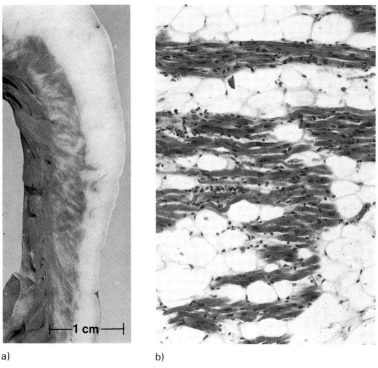

a)   b)

Fig. 6.31 a) Fat cell permeation of right ventricular wall. b) Fat cell permeation of myocardium. HE staining.

Fig. 6.32 Myocardial amyloidosis.
Congo red staining/polarized light.

6.6.5 Löeffler's endocarditis

The heart may be affected by any disease in which there is an eosinophilia. The most common cause is the hypereosinophilic syndrome, which is an idiopathic condition. Other causes include Hodgkin's disease, parasitic infections and neoplasms.

Clinically, the patient is usually young and presents with symptoms and signs of congestive heart failure. Prognosis is poor and treatment is supportive.

6.6.6 Secondary degenerative cardiomyopathies

Degenerative cardiomyopathies are forms of secondary cardiomyopathy arising as a result of the toxic action of a harmful agent, or the accumulation of specific substances due to a metabolic disorder. There are many conditions which may affect the myocardium. Usually the systolic function of the ventricle is impaired; however, diastolic dysfunction, similar to restrictive cardiomyopathy, can occur in amyloidosis or the carcinoid syndrome.

Haemochromatosis and haemosiderosis

Both these conditions result in excessive iron deposition in the heart, which causes a dilated, poorly contracting heart (see Fig. 6.35).

Amyloidosis

Cardiac amyloidosis is rare and the diagnosis can be made by endomyocardial biopsy. This complication

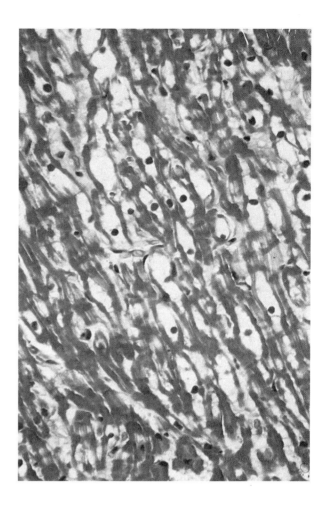

Fig. 6.33 Type II glycogenosis. Copious glycogen in the cytoplasm (optically empty myocytes after paraffin embedding). HE staining.

of amyloid has a very poor prognosis. The ECG shows low ventricular voltages. Microscopic examination of cardiac tissue reveals a deposition of amyloid diffusely between muscle fibres, surrounding blood vessels and infiltrating the conducting system (Fig. 6.32). The cardiac infiltration with amyloid impairs the diastolic filling of the ventricles.

Sarcoidosis

Infiltration of the heart by sarcoid granulomata may

result in conduction abnormalities, arrhythmias and congestive heart failure.

Alcohol

Excessive alcohol intake may cause:

1. Alcoholic cardiomyopathy.
2. Cobalt toxicity.
3. Poor dietary intake, associated with alcohol abuse, may result in beri-beri.

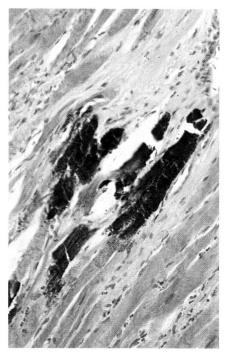

Fig. 6.34 Calcinosis. Dark brown calcium deposits in the myocardium. Kossa silvering.

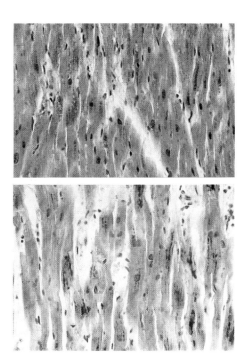

Fig. 6.35 Secondary haemochromatosis.
Above: HE staining. Below: Prussian blue reaction.

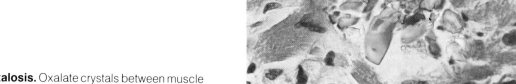

Fig. 6.36 Oxalosis. Oxalate crystals between muscle fibres in an HE stain, viewed under polarized light.

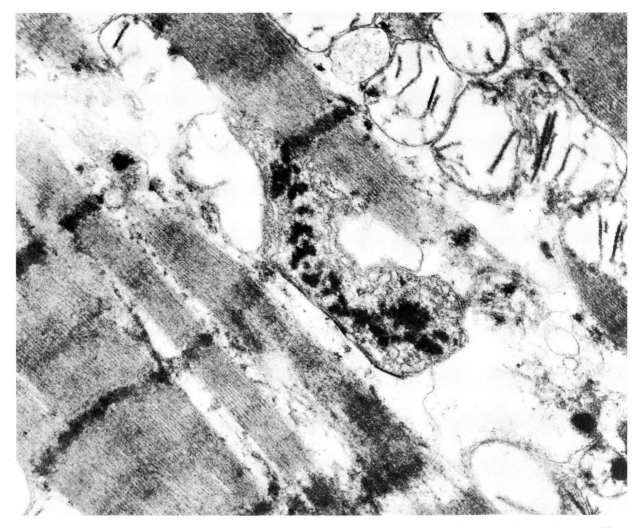

Fig. 6.37 Adriamycin cardiomyopathy. Electron micrograph of degenerative muscle fibre, with bizarrely deformed Z bands with partial lysis of fibril bundles and multiplication and swelling of mitochondria. (Tissue obtained 8h post-mortem.) Magnification ×26 500.

Cytotoxic drug therapy

The cytotoxic drugs doxorubicin, daunorubicin, adriamycin (Figs 6.37–6.38) and cyclophosphamide may all cause congestive heart failure. During treatment with these agents, patients should have their left ventricular ejection fractions monitored.

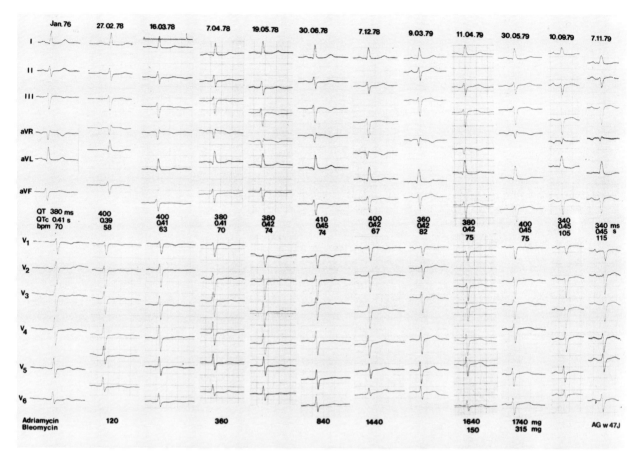

Fig. 6.38 ECG modifications during adriamycin therapy. The doses of adriamycin and bleomycin are shown. The times of administration and the heart rate determined from the ECG (bpm), with QT interval and frequency-corrected QT interval (QTc) are shown. During the course of treatment there is a rotation of the QRS vector to the left (V.a. left anterior hemiblock), sinus tachycardia and QTc prolongation as expressions of extensive myocardial injury.

6.7 MYOCARDITIS

Myocarditis is an inflammation of the myocytes and interstitial tissue with or without vasculitis.

Clinical features are variable and depend on the severity of myocardial impairment. Patients may be asymptomatic or they may have arrhythmias, congestive heart failure, or sudden death.

The pathological features vary, depending on the severity of the myocarditis and its aetiology. An inflammatory infiltrate is seen on microscopy, and myocyte necrosis, granulomata or abscesses may also be seen.

6.7.1   Viral myocarditis

Viral myocarditis is the most common cause of myocarditis in industrialized societies, and the Coxsackie B virus is the most frequent aetiological organism.

6.7.2   Bacterial myocarditis

Diphtheria

Diphtheria bacteria produce a toxin which causes myocardial necrosis, which may result in death.

Streptococcus

Beta haemolytic Group A streptococci induce an auto-immune response which can affect the myocardium. The pathological features include Aschoff nodule, which consists of a central area of fibrinoid degeneration surrounded by lympocytes, monocytes and leucocytes.

The heart can also be infected by the following bacteria: staphylococci, pneumococci, tubercle bacilli and spirochaetes.

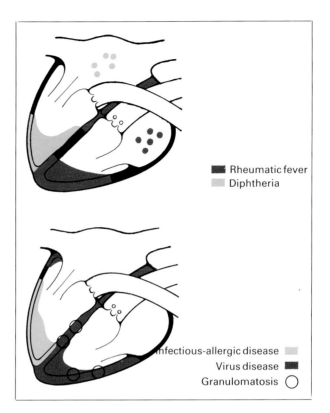

Rheumatic fever
Diphtheria

infectious-allergic disease
Virus disease
Granulomatosis

Fig. 6.39 Diagram of sites of myocarditis.

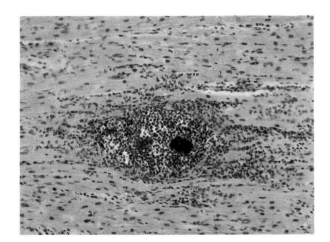

Fig. 6.40 Septic focus in the myocardium. Collection of segmented leucocytes with encapsulated bacteria. HE staining.

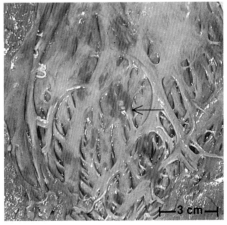

Fig. 6.41 Subendocardial pyaemic abscess (arrow) in septicaemia.

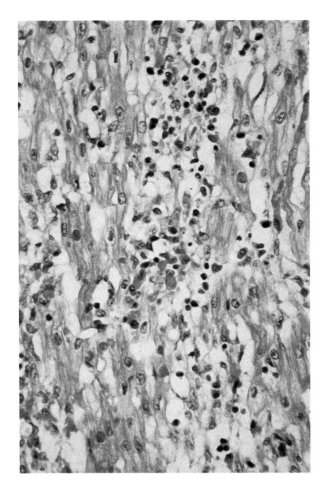

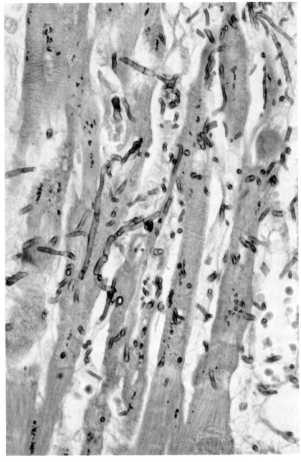

Fig. 6.42 Coxsackie myocarditis. Degradation of myocytes and dense round-cell infiltration of interstitial tissue. HE staining.

Fig. 6.43 Candida myocarditis. Numerous mycelia revealed by Grocott staining.

6.7.3 Fungal myocarditis

Candidal myocarditis (Fig. 6.43) may occur in patients who are immuno-suppressed. Other fungal infections, such as blastomyocosis or crypto-coccosis, may occur. The hyphae are easily over-looked in HE stained material but can be demons-trated selectively by PAS or Grocott staining.

6.7.4 Parasitic myocarditis

Chaga's disease is common in South America and is caused by *Trypanosoma cruzi*. Initially, the parasite invades the myocardium (Fig. 6.44), causing acute myocarditis. Most patients recover from this but many years later, congestive heart failure may develop. In the acute phase, there are numerous pseudocysts in the myocytes, with only a slight cellular reaction in the interstitial tissue. In the chronic phase of the disease, myocardial fibres are replaced by scar tissue and this is manifested clinically by congestive heart failure and cardiac hypertrophy.

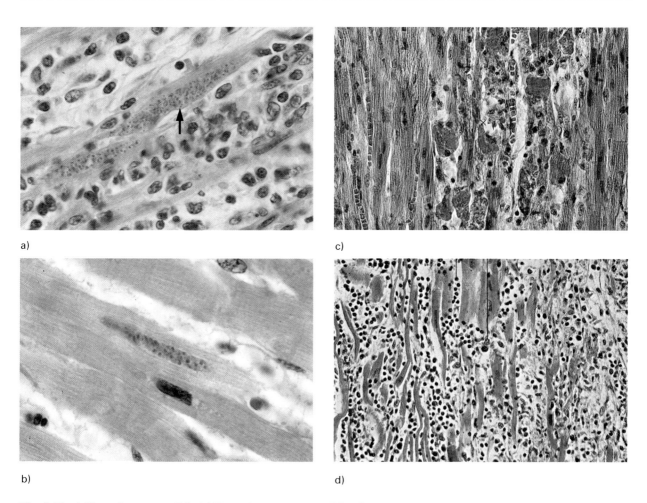

a)

c)

b)

d)

Fig. 6.44 a) Chaga's myocarditis. b) Toxoplasma myocarditis. c) Parenchymatous myocarditis in diphtheria. d) Interstitial myocarditis in scarlet fever. HE staining.

6.8 ENDOCARDITIS

Endocarditis is classified into two broad groups:

1. Infective endocarditis
2. Non-infective endocarditis

Infective endocarditis is classified by describing the infecting organism and is more common than non-infective endocarditis.

Non-infective endocarditis refers to the presence of sterile vegetations within the heart. Non-infective endocarditis occurs in rheumatic fever, terminal malignancy, systemic lupus erythematosus and carcinoid syndrome. Vegetations may be seen on echocardiography and may embolize.

6.8.1 Rheumatic fever

Acute rheumatic fever mainly occurs in young people. It is now a rare disease in industrialized societies but is still common in developing countries. Previously, rheumatic fever was the most common cause of heart disease in Britain. Although acute rheumatic fever is rare, there are still many elderly patients with cardiac complications from their acute rheumatic fever when they were children.

Rheumatic fever is caused by Group A haemolytic streptococcal throat infection. This induces antibody formation which cross-reacts with the patient's own cells, causing damage. The pathological features of rheumatic fever are due to an

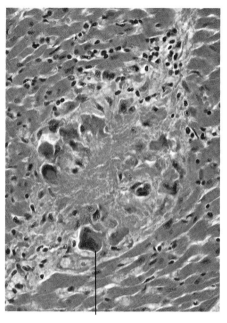

Fig. 6.46 Aschoff's granuloma in rheumatic myocarditis. Numerous Aschoff's cells (↑). HE staining.

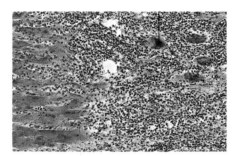

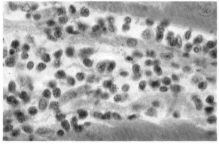

Fig. 6.47 Above: **Giant cell myocarditis.** Below: **Fiedler's myocarditis** with eosinophilic granulocytes. HE staining.

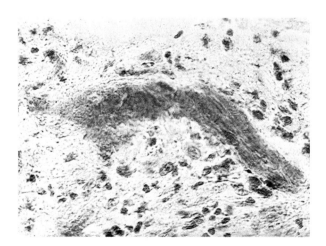

Fig. 6.45 Rheumatic myocarditis. Fresh fibrinoid necrosis. HE staining.

inflammatory response affecting connective tissue (Fig. 6.45). The connective tissue involved is in the heart, joints and skin. The inflammatory response eventually results in Aschoff nodules (Fig. 6.46), which are pathognomonic of rheumatic fever. The inflammatory reaction involving the heart affects the pericardium, myocardium and, most commonly, the endocardium. Inflammation of the endocardium over the cardiac valves results in oedematous nodules. Subsequent fibrosis of the inflamed tissues can cause deformity of the heart valves. The leaflets may adhere to each other, causing valvular stenosis, or they become fibrosed and shortened, causing valvular incompetence. The progression from acute rheumatic fever to chronic valvular dysfunction occurs over many years and there are usually repeated attacks of rheumatic fever.

Acute rheumatic fever

A steptococcal throat infection is followed 7–35 days later by the following symptoms and signs. To make the diagnosis of rheumatic fever, evidence of a preceding streptococcal throat infection, plus either two major criteria or one major plus two minor criteria, should be present.

Major criteria
Carditis
Arthritis
Chorea
Subcutaneous nodules
Erythema marginatum

Minor criteria
Fever
Arthralgia
Previous rheumatic fever
Raised acute phase reactions
Prolonged PR interval

The acute attack of rheumatic fever usually settles within three months. Further streptococcal throat infection will cause further attacks of rheumatic fever which can progress to chronic rheumatic valvular disease, which is the most important complication of rheumatic fever.

6.8.2 Bacterial endocarditis

Subacute endocarditis

Subacute endocarditis usually presents with a chronic low-grade pyrexia, anorexia, weight loss

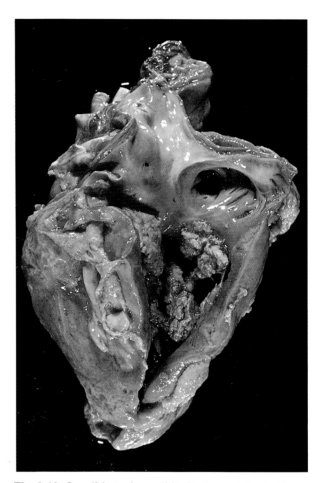

Fig. 6.48 Candida endocarditis. Right heart filled with large, grey-brown fungal mass.

and a heart murmur. It is usually caused by a less virulent organism than acute endocarditis and there is usually an underlying cardiac abnormality which predisposes to subacute endocarditis. The prognosis is good if the illness is recognized and treated adequately. Organisms, such as *Streptococcus viridans*, *Streptococcus faecalis*, *Staphylococcus epidermis*, *Rickettsia*, fungi, *E. coli* and *Pseudomonas*, may all cause subacute endocarditis.

Acute endocarditis

Acute endocarditis usually presents with a high pyrexia, murmur and rapidly progressive heart failure. It is usually caused by a virulent organism and there need not be any underlying cardiac disease. There is rapid destruction of the cardiac tissue by the virulent organism and the prognosis is poor. Organisms, such as *Staphylococcus aureus* and *Pneumococcus* may cause acute endocarditis.

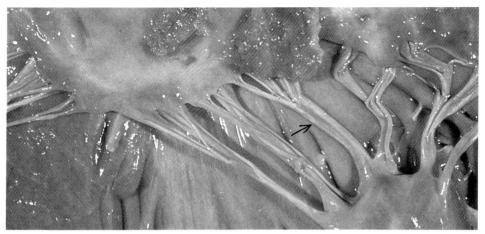

Fig. 6.49 Nonbacterial, verrucous endocarditis in rheumatic fever. Arrow = thickened tendon strands.

Subacute endocarditis

The initial lesion in this condition is the sterile vegetation, which develops in areas of turbulent blood flow within the heart. The vegetation consists of platelets and fibrin. Pre-existing cardiac lesions, such as congenital heart disease or rheumatic valvular disease, predispose to vegetation formation. If micro-organisms are released into the blood stream, they can colonize the vegetations, making it an infected vegetation.

Cardiac lesions predisposing to bacterial endocarditis:

Aortic valve disease
Mitral valve disease
Coarctation of the aorta
Patent ductus arteriosus
Ventricular septal defect
Prosthetic valves
Pacemaker
Hypertrophic cardiomyopathy

Mild valvular lesions are more prone to infection than severe valve lesions.

Bacterial endocarditis can present with a wide variety of symptoms and signs, which relate to:

1. Symptoms and signs of chronic infection.
2. Symptoms and signs of cardiac disease.
3. Symptoms and signs of embolic phenomenon.
4. Symptoms and signs of an immune response.

The infective symptoms and signs include fever, myalgia, arthralgia, malaise, loss of weight, anaemia, clubbing and splenomegaly.

The cardiac features include symptoms and signs of congestive heart failure, new murmurs or sudden haemodynamic deterioration due to acute endocarditis eroding a valve.

Emboli may break off and occlude an artery, which may result in abscess formation. Common sites of embolization include the brain, eyes, kidneys, femoral and mesenteric arteries.

The immune response to chronic infection results in high levels of circulating immune complexes. These can cause a vasculitis or glomerulonephritis. Clinically, the immune reaction can manifest as a rash, splinter haemorrhages, Roth spots or renal impairment, with haematuria and proteinuria.

Investigations

Six blood cultures should be taken to attempt to identify the infecting organism. Haematological findings in subacute bacterial endocarditis include a raised ESR, anaemia, leucocytosis and a raised CRP.

Echocardiography
Echocardiography may confirm the clinical diagnosis but a negative echo cannot exclude bacterial endocarditis because the vegetations may be too small to be seen.

Other investigations that should be performed include urea and electrolytes, chest X-ray, ECG and urinalysis. These investigations may give evidence of specific complications arising from subacute bacterial endocarditis.

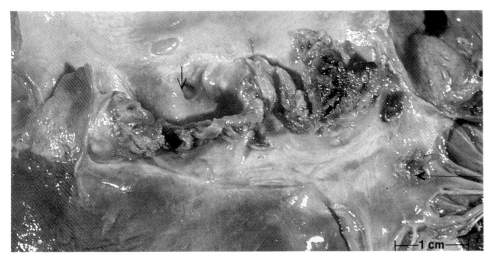

Fig. 6.50 Acute bacterial, ulcerative endocarditis.
(↓ coronary ostium; ← mitral leaflet endocarditis).

Blood cultures should be taken before the commencement of antibiotic therapy as the choice of antibiotic depends on the organism isolated from the blood and its sensitivity. Antibiotics are usually given for at least six weeks.

Acute bacterial endocarditis

Acute bacterial endocarditis is caused by virulent organisms which can attack directly normal hearts. It is a rapidly progressive disease with poor prognosis. The valves most commonly affected by endocarditis are the mitral and aortic valves.

The following forms of endocarditis are differentiated morphologically:

1. Verrucous endocarditis occurs mainly in rheumatic fever and malignant disease. It is characterized by delicate, reddish, readily removable deposits of platelets and fibrin (Fig. 6.49).
2. Ulcerative endocarditis involves an extensive destruction of the valves and occurs mainly in acute infective endocarditis.
3. Polypous endocarditis: these are large vegetations composed of erythrocytes, leucocytes, fibrin, platelets and bacteria. The underlying valves often exhibit extensive damage and this occurs mainly with subacute endocarditis. Particularly large vegetations are found in fungal endocarditis which, unlike the other forms of endocarditis, may also be located on the right side of the heart.

Non-infective endocarditis

Non-infective endocarditis may occur in:

Rheumatic fever
Malignancy (Marantic endocarditis)
Systemic lupus erythematosus (Libmann-Sach's endocarditis)

Carcinoid syndrome
In the carcinoid syndrome, the valves on the right side of the heart are predominantly affected. The valves and right ventricle become fibrosed, causing symptoms and signs of right ventricular failure.

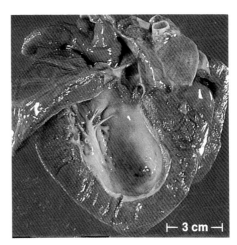

Fig. 6.51 Endocardial fibrosis.

6.9 ACQUIRED HEART VALVE DEFECTS

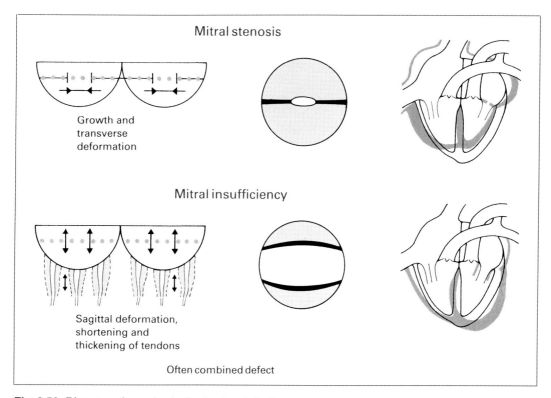

Fig. 6.52 Diagram of acquired mitral valve defects.

Heart valve defects are defined as organic or functional valvular disorders which may cause valvular stenosis or incompetence. In organic valvular disease there are alterations in structure of the valve itself. The cusps may be incompetent or they may adhere to each other, causing stenosis. Functional valve defects are the result of dilatation of the valvular ring and/or displacement of the papillary muscles, so that the valve cusps can no longer close but the valves themselves are normal. In congestive heart failure, ventricular dilatation may distort the mitral valve apparatus causing mitral regurgitation.

6.9.1 Mitral stenosis

Mitral stenosis is most commonly due to rheumatic fever. Mitral stenosis occurs more commonly in females than in males, the ratio being 3 : 1. Mitral stenosis can occasionally occur as an isolated congenital lesion or in association with other congenital defects such as an atrial septal defect. (This is called Lutembacher's syndrome.)

The normal size of a mitral valve orifice is 6cm^2. In severe mitral stenosis, the orifice is less than 1cm^2. Mitral stenosis impairs left ventricular filling and this causes raised left atrial, pulmonary vein and pulmonary capillary wedge pressures.

Pathology

Rheumatic fever causes inflammation of the mitral valve cusps and eventually the valve cusps may adhere to each other, reducing the mitral valve orifice (Figs 6.53 and 6.54). Mitral stenosis impedes blood flow through the mitral valve, which causes stasis of the blood in the left atrium. This predisposes to thrombus formation.

Clinical features

A patient with mitral stenosis may complain of the following symptoms: dyspnoea, haemoptysis, fatigue, palpitations, symptoms of right ventricular failure, or chest pain. The patient may also describe symptoms due to arterial emboli and the symptoms relate to the site of the embolus. Examination of a patient with mitral stenosis may reveal a malar flush, signs of right ventricular failure, pulmonary oedema, atrial fibrillation, tapping apex beat or signs of arterial embolization. The auscultatory findings of mitral stenosis depend on the valvular leaflet mobility but usually the first heart sound is loud and an opening snap is heard after the second heart sound. A low-pitched rumbling diastolic murmur follows the opening snap. The severity of mitral stenosis is indicated by the duration of the diastolic murmur, not its loudness.

ECG

The ECG may show atrial fibrillation and if the patient is in sinus rhythm, P mitrale. Right ventricular hypertrophy and right axis deviation occur if pulmonary hypertension has developed.

Chest X-ray

The chest X-ray may show a large left atrium, pulmonary oedema, calcified mitral valve and widened carina. If pulmonary hypertension develops, right ventricular hypertrophy and large pulmonary arteries are seen.

Echocardiography

The echocardiogram will show reduced movement of the anterior mitral valve cusp, parallel movement of the anterior and posterior mitral valve leaflets, reduced diastolic closure rate, calcification of the mitral valve leaflets or annulus, large left atrium and normal-sized left ventricle.

6.9.2   Mitral regurgitation

Mitral regurgitation may result from abnormalities of the mitral valve leaflets, chordae tendineae or papillary muscles (organic valve disease). Functional mitral regurgitation may occur due to dilatation of the mitral valve annulus due to left ventricular dilatation. Mitral regurgitation allows blood to flow back into the left atrium during systole. The left atrial pressure may rise, causing a raised pulmonary capillary wedge pressure and pulmonary oedema. Acute mitral regurgitation may present with cardiogenic shock and pulmonary oedema and usually occurs post myocardial infarction. The left atrium is not compliant and is unable to compensate for the acute volume load placed upon it. In chronic mitral regurgitation, the left atrium has had time to hypertrophy and compensate for the excess volume load which is placed upon it by the mitral regurgitation. Chronic mitral regurgita-

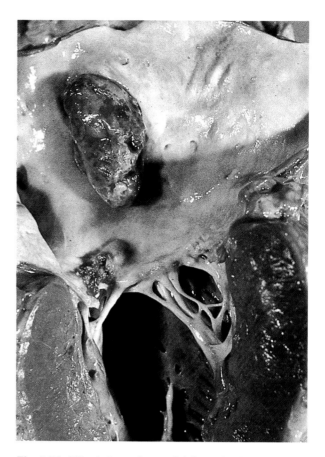

Fig. 6.53 Mitral stenosis—atrial thrombosis. Previous scarring due to rheumatic endocarditis with shortened, plump tendon cords and marked valve thickening. A ball thrombus adherent to the wall is present in the atrium.

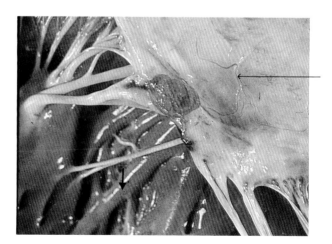

Fig. 6.54 Recurrent rheumatic mitral endocarditis. (Arrow: vascularization of mitral flap). ↓ : Trabeculum.

tion presents with symptoms of congestive heart failure. Mitral regurgitation causes a blowing pansystolic murmur, loudest at the apex and radiating to the axilla. Other signs are dependent upon the severity of the mitral regurgitation.

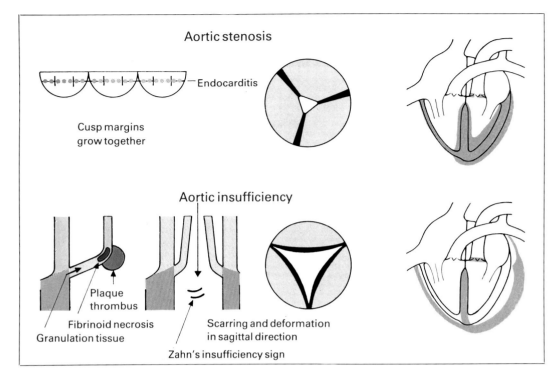

Fig. 6.55 Diagram of acquired aortic valve defects.

Causes

Organic

1. Rheumatic fever
2. Papillary muscle rupture (MI)
3. Sub-acute bacterial endocarditis
4. Marfan's syndrome
5. Congenital heart disease

Functional
Left ventricular dilatation, e.g. cardiomyopathy.

ECG

The ECG may show signs of left ventricular hypertrophy, strain or left axis deviation.

Chest X-ray

The chest X-ray may show evidence of left ventricular hypertrophy, left atrial hypertrophy or pulmonary oedema.

Echocardiography

The echocardiogram may show a prolapsing mitral valve leaflet and allows chamber size to be assessed. Chamber size depends on the severity and duration of the mitral regurgitation.

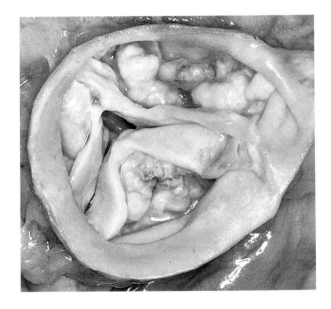

Fig. 6.56 Aortic valve stenosis due to arteriosclerosis.
Margins of cusps largely free, with arteriosclerotic vegetations deeper down.

6.9.3 Mitral valve prolapse

This condition is due to mucopolysaccharide deposition in the zona spongiosa of the valve leaflets. This causes weakening of the valve leaflets, which can stretch and prolapse. This condition affects up to 2% of healthy people and is more

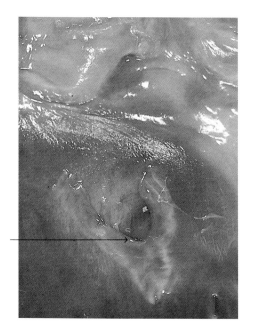

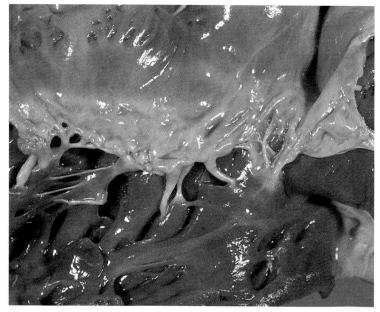

Fig. 6.57 Zahn's insufficiency sign.
Pseudovalve (→) in the endocardium of
the outflow tract of the left ventricle in aortic
valve regurgitation.

Fig. 6.58 Tricuspid thickening in the carcinoid syndrome.

common in females than in males. Most patients are completely asymptomatic, the murmur being found during a routine examination. Symptoms which may occur due to mitral valve prolapse include palpitations and chest pain. Rarely, complications, such as systemic emboli or progressive mitral regurgitation, may develop. Examination reveals a mid to late systolic murmur and other signs, such as those of congestive heart failure, depend on the severity of the mitral regurgitation.

The ECG is usually normal but may have non-specific ST-T wave changes. The echocardiogram will show evidence of mitral valve prolapse. Mitral valve prolapse can also occur in several connective tissue diseases, such as Marfan's syndrome or Ehlers-Danlos syndrome.

6.9.4 Aortic valve stenosis

The normal aortic valve orifice is 5cm². In aortic stenosis, the orifice is reduced in size, which causes obstruction of the left ventricular outflow tract. Aortic stenosis may be due to a congenital abnormality, senile valve calcification or rheumatic valve disease. Aortic stenosis may be asymptomatic or it may cause symptoms of congestive heart failure, angina or syncope. Examination may reveal a displaced apex beat, small volume and slow-rising pulse. On auscultation of the heart, a harsh ejection

systolic murmur is heard over the aortic area, which may radiate to the carotids and the aortic component of the second heart sound is quiet. The ECG may show evidence of left ventricular hypertrophy, left axis deviation or left bundle branch block.

Chest X-ray

The chest X-ray may show evidence of left ventricular hypertrophy, calcified aortic valve and post-stenotic dilatation of the aorta. Signs of left ventricular failure may also be seen.

Echocardiography

The echocardiogram shows a calcified valve with a narrow orifice. Left ventricular hypertrophy is also seen.

Aortic stenosis has a poor prognosis once it becomes symptomatic. Death usually occurs from left ventricular failure, arrhythmias or myocardial infarction.

6.9.5 Aortic valve regurgitation

This may be due to an abnormality of the valve allowing blood to leak back through the aortic valve in diastole, or it may be due to dilatation of the

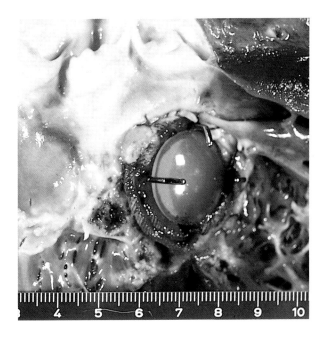

Fig. 6.59 Mitral replacement by Starr-Edwards ball prosthesis.

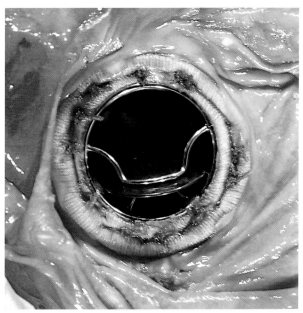

Fig. 6.60 Mitral replacement by Shilley butterfly prosthesis. View in the atrium.

aortic root separating the normal valve cusps from their closure lines, allowing diastolic leakage. The regurgitant jet causes left ventricular dilatation and left ventricular hypertrophy. Over time, the left ventricular function may deteriorate and heart failure result.

Causes

Valve lesions
Rheumatic fever
Sub-acute bacterial endocarditis
Congenital abnormalities of the valve
Rheumatoid arthritis
Aortic root disease
Aortic dissection
Syphilis
Marfan's syndrome
Trauma
Ankylosing spondylitis
Reiter's syndrome
Hypertension

The patient with aortic regurgitation may complain of symptoms suggestive of congestive heart failure but aortic regurgitation is commonly asymptomatic. Examination may reveal signs of an underlying disorder and aortic regurgitation itself causes a collapsing pulse, displaced apex beat and an early diastolic murmur which is heard best at the left sternal edge when the patient sits forward and holds his breath at the end of expiration.

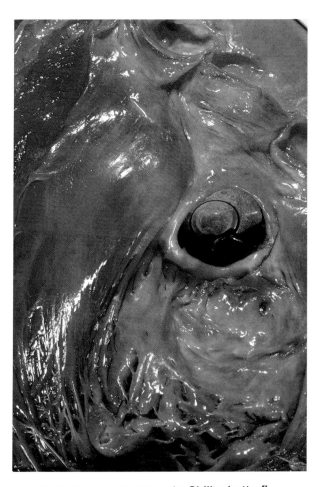

Fig. 6.61 Mitral replacement by Shilley butterfly prosthesis. View in the left ventricle.

ECG

The ECG may show evidence of left ventricular hypertrophy, left axis deviation or left bundle branch block.

Chest X-ray

The chest X-ray may show signs of left ventricular hypertrophy, aortic dilatation and aortic valve calcification.

Echocardiography

The echocardiogram demonstrates the size of the left ventricle and its function. The aortic regurgitation is seen on the echo as fluttering of the anterior mitral leaflet in diastole. The aortic valve may be thickened and calcified and the size of the aortic root can also be assessed.

Prognosis

The prognosis for patients is poor once they develop symptoms from their aortic regurgitation.

6.9.6 Tricuspid stenosis

This valvular lesion is usually due to rheumatic fever and is accompanied by mitral and aortic valvular disease. Tricuspid stenosis impairs filling of the right ventricle, causing raised right atrial pressure and venous congestion.

6.9.7 Tricuspid regurgitation

Tricuspid regurgitation is usually functional rather than organic in origin. It is commonly associated with conditions which cause right ventricular hypertrophy, such as pulmonary hypertension, cor pulmonale and cardiomyopathies. The organic causes of tricuspid regurgitation include bacterial endocarditis, rheumatic fever, carcinoid syndrome and trauma. It is unusual for bacterial endocarditis to affect the valves on the right side of the heart but this does occur in drug addicts who repeatedly inject themselves intravenously with dirty needles. Emboli from the tricuspid valve may cause repeated pulmonary infarctions which may become abscesses. This may be the presenting feature of a patient with right-sided bacterial endocarditis.

6.9.8 Pulmonary stenosis

Pulmonary stenosis obstructs the right ventricular outflow tract and is usually due to a congenital disorder.

6.9.9 Pulmonary regurgitation

Pulmonary regurgitation is a very rare organic valvular defect.

6.9.10 Heart valve replacement

Heart valve replacement (Figs 6.59–6.61) involves replacing the aortic, mitral or, rarely, the right heart valves, with artificial valves which can be either mechanical or prosthetic. The complications of valve replacement include:

1. Valve failure. The artificial valve fails structurally, which causes valvular regurgitation and haemodynamic deterioration.
2. Endocarditis may occur in artificial valves.
3. Thrombo-embolism.
4. Suture dehiscence. This can cause a para-valvular leak and haemodynamic deterioration.
5. Haemolysis.

6.10 CONGENITAL HEART DISEASE

Definition

Congenital heart defects are the macroscopic abnormalities of the heart present from birth.

The incidence of congenital heart defects is 8/1000 live births in the UK. Congenital heart defects are due to a combination of genetic and environmental factors, a multi-factorial aetiology. The heart defect in an individual patient may be either primarily chromosomal in origin or there may be a known environmental factor, but in most cases it is presumed that the cardiac defect is due to a combination of genetic and environmental factors. Chromosomal disorders which may cause congenital heart disease include Down's syndrome, Turner's syndrome and Marfan's syndrome. Environmental factors which can affect the mother and cause fetal cardiac abnormalities include alcohol abuse, rubella infection or thalidomide ingestion.

Clinical features

The clinical features of congenital heart disease range from asymptomatic heart conditions detected on routine examination, to life-threatening illnesses. The clinical findings depend on the defect, its severity and whether or not the defect is part of a syndrome or an isolated lesion.

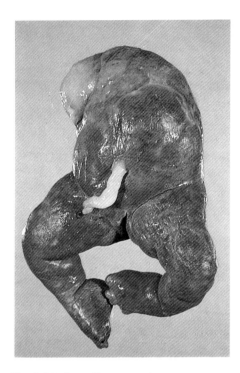

Fig. 6.62 Acardius amorphus.

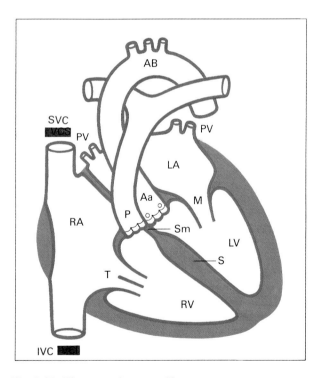

Fig. 6.63 Diagram of a normal heart.

RA:	right atrium,	M:	mitral valve,
T:	tricuspid valve,	LV:	left ventricle,
RV:	right ventricle,	Aa:	ascending aorta,
S:	septum,	AB:	aortic arch,
Sm:	membranous septum,	SVC:	superior vena cava,
P:	pulmonary artery,	IVC:	inferior vena cava,
LA:	left atrium,	PV:	pulmonary veins.

Classification

1. Congenital heart defects without shunts
   Heart valve defects
   Coarctation of the aorta
2. Congenital heart defects with primary left-to-right shunt
   Atrial septal defect
   Ventricular septal defect
   Patent ductus arteriosus
3. Congenital heart defects with primary right-to-left shunt (cyanosis)
   Truncus arteriosus communis
   Transposition of the great arteries
   Fallot's tetralogy
   Tricuspid atresia
   Total anomalous pulmonary venous drainage
   Double outlet right ventricle
   Eisenmenger's syndrome

Congenital heart defects may obstruct blood flow, cause shunting of blood from the left side of the heart to the right side (acyanotic heart defect) and cause shunting of blood from the right side of the heart to the left side of the heart (cyanotic heart disease).

Normally, pressures on the left side of the heart are greater than those on the right and if a shunt is present, blood is shunted from left to right. However, if the pressure on the right side of the heart is greater than the pressure on the left, blood will flow from the right to the left side.

A left-to-right shunt increases the pulmonary blood flow and may result in pulmonary hypertension. With time, the pressure on the right side of the heart will increase and may become greater than the pressure on the left side of the heart. Thus, the direction of the shunt may change from left to right, to right to left. An acyanotic shunt may cause pulmonary hypertension and the shunt reverses causing cyanosis.

Complications of congenital heart disease include heart failure, endocarditis, thrombo-embolism, cerebral abscesses and sudden death.

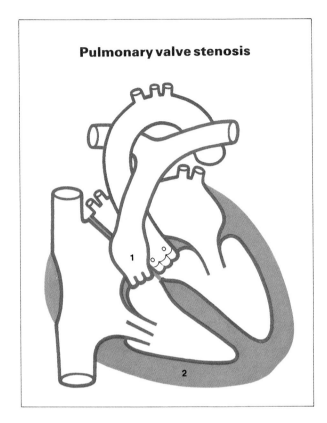

Pulmonary valve stenosis

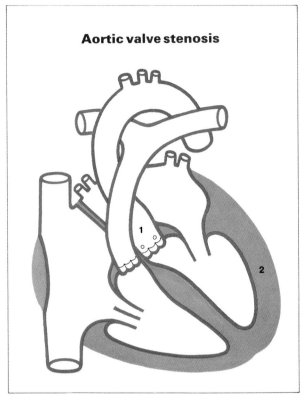

Aortic valve stenosis

Fig. 6.64 Congenital pulmonary valve stenosis with suprastenotic dilatation (1) and hypertrophy of the right ventricular wall (2).

Fig. 6.65 Congenital aortic valve stenosis with suprastenotic dilatation (1) and hypertrophy of the left ventricular wall.

Incidence of cardiovascular malformation

Cardiovascular malformations	Incidence	Lethality
1. Ventricular septal defect (VSD)	30%	–
2. Atrial septal defect (ASD)	10%	–
3. Patent ductus arteriosus (PDA)	10%	20%
4. Pulmonary stenosis (PS)	7%	10%
5. Coarctation of aorta	7%	
Preductal infantile form		89%
Postductal adult form		60%
6. Aortic stenosis	6%	10%
7. Fallot's tetralogy	6%	30%
8. Complete transposition	4%	90%
9. Truncus arteriosus communis	2%	–
10. Tricuspid atresia	1%	66%
11. Other malformations	17%	–

Congenital heart defects may occur either in isolation or as part of a complex cardiovascular malformation.

6.10.1   Pulmonary stenosis

Pulmonary stenosis usually occurs at the valvular level but can be either supra- or infra-valvular. In valvular pulmonary stenosis, there is narrowing of the valve with post stenotic dilatation.

Sub-valvular infundibular stenosis is a component of Fallot's tetralogy and is only rarely an isolated defect.

Supra-valvular pulmonary stenosis causes a pressure load on the right ventricle and thus right ventricular hypertrophy.

The murmur of pulmonary stenosis is a harsh ejection systolic murmur best heard over the pulmonary area. Most children with pulmonary stenosis are asymptomatic and the prognosis in this condition is good if the pressure gradient across the valve is less than 25mmHg.

6.10.2   Aortic stenosis

Approximately 70% of aortic stenoses are valvular in origin (Fig. 6.65), whereas the supra- and infra-valvular forms each comprise 15%. Aortic stenosis occurs predominantly in males, with a ratio of 4 : 1. In valvular stenosis there is fusion of the commissures: the valve ring may be of normal width or narrowed. The supra-valvular and infra-valvular

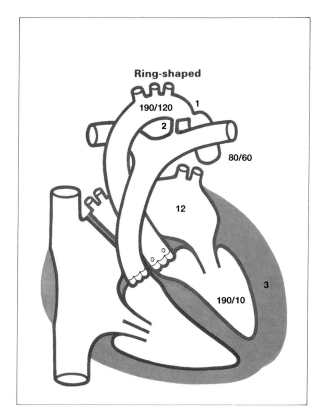
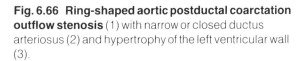

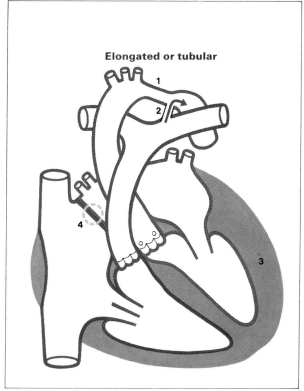

Fig. 6.66 Ring-shaped aortic postductal coarctation outflow stenosis (1) with narrow or closed ductus arteriosus (2) and hypertrophy of the left ventricular wall (3).

Fig. 6.67 Elongated or tubular **aortic preductal coarctation outflow stenosis** (1) in front of the open ductus arteriosus (2). Hypertrophy of the left ventricular wall (3). There is frequently also an atrial septal defect (4).

forms of aortic stenosis are caused by a membranous structure which impairs the blood flow in the left ventricular outflow tract. All forms of aortic stenoses cause a pressure load on the left ventricle. Pressure gradients across the stenoses of 80mmHg or greater, or if the valve orifice is less than $0.5cm^2/m^2$ body surface area, indicate the stenosis is severe.

6.10.3 Coarctation of the aorta

The aortic isthmus is the area where the aortic arch becomes the descending aorta, immediately after the origin of the left subclavian artery. Stenoses here may be circumscribed or diffuse. A bicuspid aortic valve occurs as a concomitant malformation in 50% of cases. A 60% narrowing of the aorta induces the formation of a collateral circulation between the subclavian arteries, internal thoracic, intercostal and internal mammary arteries. Rib notching involving the lower margin of the ribs 4–8 can be seen on chest X-ray as a consequence of

dilated intercostal arteries. The main clinical findings are raised blood pressure in the arms and low blood pressure in the legs, radio-femoral delay on palpation of the pulses, a continuous murmur heard best over the thoracic spine or below the left clavicle and visible pulsation over the scapulae with a continuous bruit if a collateral circulation has developed. The complications of aortic coarctation include cerebral haemorrhage, dissection of aortic aneurysm, heart failure, bacterial endocarditis and persistent hypertension, even after surgical correction of the aortic coarctation.

Two types of aortic isthmus stenosis are distinguished.

a) Adult type
The coarctation is due to an isolated membranous lesion located either immediately in the area of an already obliterated ductus arteriosus or slightly post ductal. The coarctation develops slowly and the patient usually presents between 15 and 30 years of age with complications. The mean life expectancy of these patients is 35 years.

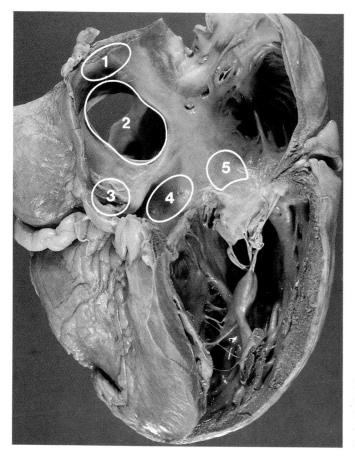

Fig. 6.68 Atrial septal defect (ostium secundum defect). Photograph of the opened right heart with tricuspid valve. 1: superior sinus venosus defect. 2: ostium secundum defect. 3: inferior sinus venosus defect. 4: coronary sinus defect.

b) Infantile type

In the infantile type, the coarctation is situated pre ductally and the ductus arteriosus is patent. Venous blood from the pulmonary artery mixes with aortic blood. The prognosis is poor with this form of aortic coarctation and the mean survival time is less than 1 year.

6.10.4 Pseudo-coarctation

An elongated aorta (Fig. 6.67) is kinked in the area of the ligamentum arteriosum but not constricted, so there are normal blood pressures in all four limbs. This is of no haemodynamic significance.

6.10.5 Atrial septal defect (ASD)

ASD (Fig. 6.68) is the fourth most common congenital heart defect in children and is frequently diagnosed first in adult life. It affects females more commonly than males with a ratio of 2 : 1. ASDs can occur in isolation or in combination with other abnormalities, e.g. mitral stenosis and ASD Lutembacher's syndrome. ASD plus upper limb bony deformities Holt-Oram's syndrome.

The condition to be distinguished from an ASD is an incompletely closed foramen ovale, which can be detected in 20–35% of all autopsy cases. Under normal physiological conditions there is no mixing of venous and arterial blood even with an anatomically open foramen ovale (Fig. 6.69), because a thin flap on the left atrial side is pressed against the foramen ovale by the higher pressure in the left atrium and thus provides a functional seal. Paradoxical embolism (Fig. 6.70) designates the passage of a thrombus from the veins of the systemic circulation into the aortic branches. It may occur in patients with a known intra-cardiac shunt or through a patent foramen ovale. Usually, the left atrial pressure exceeds the right atrial pressure and the flap is pressed against the foramen ovale, sealing it. However, if the right atrial pressure becomes greater than the left atrial pressure, the seal may no longer be intact. This could allow the passage of a thrombus from the venous circulation to pass into the left side of the heart without the presence of a known intra-cardiac shunt. The commonest cause of a raised right atrial pressure is acute cor pulmonale secondary to pulmonary emboli but it can also occur with pulmonary stenosis, COAD and pulmonary hypertension. The average of a patient with paradoxical embolism is 50 years and women are more commonly affected than men.

Pathology

The classification and morphology of ASDs are related to the embryological development of the heart.

At the beginning of the fourth week of intra-uterine life, the fetal common atrium is divided by the septum primum which grows from the dorsal and cranial parts of the atrium towards the endocardial cushions. The ostium primum refers to the foramen between the septum primum growing down and the endocardial cushions. The ostium secundum defect is due to a deficiency in the atrial septal wall. The ostium secundum defect is the most common form of ASD, namely a central, round defect that is found in the fossa ovalis. Defects of the ostium primum type are located below the fossa ovalis and are generally associated with a cleft AV valve. The ASD causes increased blood flow through the pulmonary circulation and the left side of the heart remains small in relation to the right side. Due to the increased pulmonary blood flow, a gradual increase in pulmonary artery pressure may occur.

Clinical features

A secundum ASD is usually diagnosed after the third year of life, when an asymptomatic heart murmur is detected on routine screening. Only large secundum defects cause symptoms and the child may present with dyspnoea, recurrent chest infections, wheeze, palpitations or fatigue. The clinical findings are those of right ventricular hypertrophy, and/or right ventricular failure. Auscultation of the heart reveals fixed splitting of the second heart sound and a pulmonary ejection systolic murmur due to increased pulmonary blood flow.

A secundum ASD may present for the first time in adult life with right ventricular failure, pulmonary hypertension, atrial fibrillation or paradoxical embolism. The mean life expectancy of a patient with secundum ASD is approximately 40 years.

Ostium primum defects are much less common than secundum defects and are more complex and

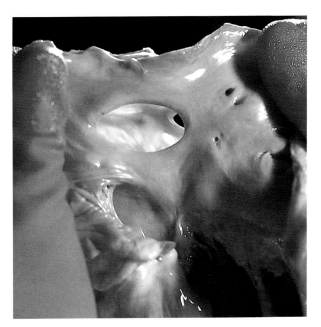

Fig. 6.69 Patent foramen ovale. Heart held against the light (viewed from the right ventricle).

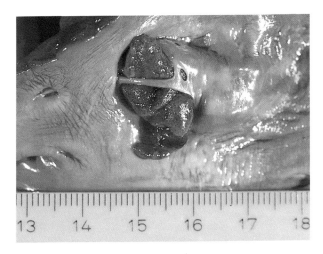

Fig. 6.70 Paradoxical embolism. Embolus in the patent foramen ovale (viewed from the right atrium).

serious, as the AV canal is also involved. Primum defects are often associated with other cardiac lesions, such as VSD or mitral regurgitation. Primum defects usually present in childhood with heart failure.

Chest X-ray

The chest X-ray of a patient with an ASD may show large pulmonary arteries, right ventricular hypertrophy and right atrial enlargement.

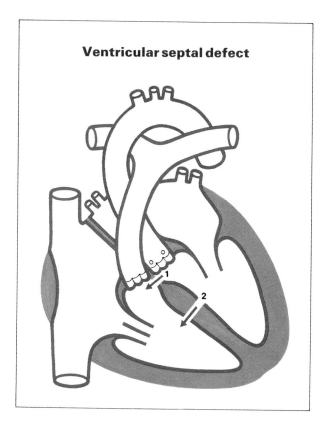

Ventricular septal defect

Fig. 6.71 **Ventricular septal defect** in the membranous septum (1) or in the muscular septum (2).

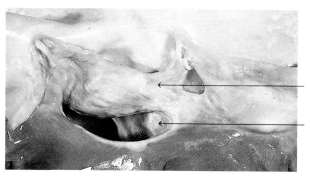

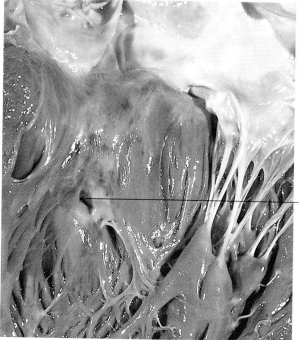

Fig. 6.72 **Above: high ventricular septal defect.** (Upper arrow: aortic valve; lower arrow: defect.) **Below: Defect in muscular septum** (arrow: defect).

ECG

The ECG of a secundum defect shows right bundle branch block and right axis deviation, whereas a primum defect shows right bundle branch block and left axis deviation.

Echocardiography

The echocardiogram may be used to demonstrate the ASD with contrast studies. The echocardiogram will also give information about the size of the right atrium and right ventricle.

Cardiac catheterization is performed to confirm the diagnosis and to assess ventricular function and pulmonary artery pressure.

6.10.6   Lutembacher's syndrome

This is a combination of an ASD and congenital or acquired mitral stenosis. Due to the elevated left atrial pressure, there is a left-to-right shunt with consequent pulmonary hypertension and right heart overload, which produces late mixed cyanosis.

6.10.7   Ventricular septal defect (VSD)

VSD is the most common form of congenital heart defect and can occur either in isolation (Fig. 6.71) or as part of a complex abnormality.

The VSD can be located in the membranous part of the septum below the valve cusps or in the muscular part of the septum (Fig. 6.72). It is not the location but the size of the VSD which is clinically important. If the VSD is large, increased pulmonary blood flow and pulmonary hypertension result. VSDs can range in size from small defects of no haemodynamic significance to large defects which

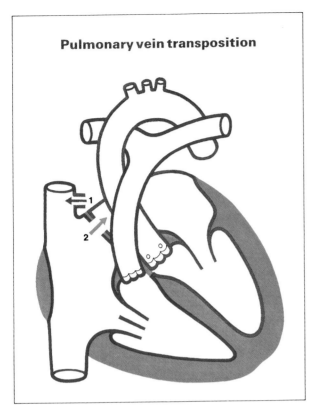

Fig. 6.73 Pulmonary vein transposition with transposition of the large veins. Incorrect opening into the superior vena cava (1) and atrial septal defect (2).

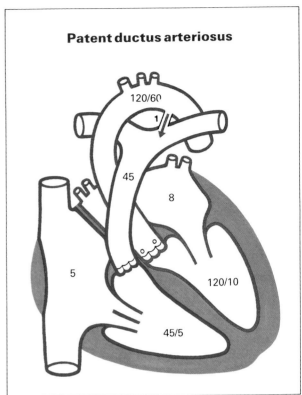

Fig. 6.74 Patent ductus arteriosus (1).

significantly raise pulmonary blood flow. The symptoms and physical signs of a patient with a VSD depend on the size of the defect.

Small VSD

The patient may be asymptomatic and a loud pansystolic murmur be detected at a routine screening examination.

Medium-sized VSD

This may present with symptoms and signs of congestive heart failure and the patient may have signs of right and/or left ventricular hypertrophy, in addition to their systolic murmur. The murmur is pansystolic, harsh and best heard at the left sternal edge.

Large VSD

A large VSD will present in the neonate with severe heart failure. Most VSDs are relatively small and some close spontaneously. Haemodynamically

significant VSDs may be complicated by heart failure, pulmonary hypertension, aortic regurgitation or Eisenmenger's syndrome. All VSDs may be complicated by bacterial endocarditis. The diagnosis is confirmed at cardiac catheterization when a step-up in the oxygen saturation is found between the right atrium and right ventricle.

6.10.8 Pulmonary vein transposition

In this condition, one (isolated form) of all four pulmonary veins (complete form) may open into the right atrium or into a vein. An ASD maintains life as mixed arterial and venous blood passes from the right atrium through to the left atrium and into the left ventricle and reaches the systemic circulation. Cyanosis develops if the transposition of the veins is total. The following forms are distinguished:

1. Supra-cardiac form (comprising 50% of all cases). Drainage into a left superior vena cava or into a right superior vena cava.
2. Cardiac form (15%). Drainage into the right

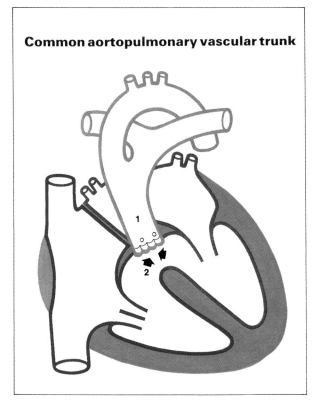

Fig. 6.75 Common aortopulmonary vascular trunk (1) with 4-cusped valve and high ventricular septal defect (2).

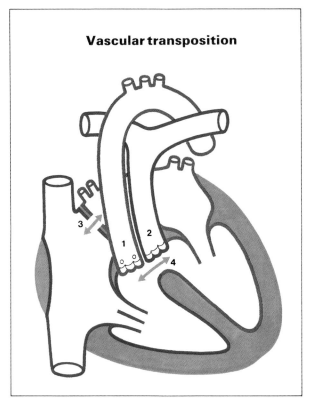

.**Fig. 6.76** Non-crossed **vascular transposition** of aorta (1) and pulmonary artery (2). Atrial (3) and ventricular septal defect (4).

atrium. In 90% of the complete pulmonary venous transposition, all four veins open into the right atrium.

3. Infra-cardiac form (15%). Drainage into the inferior vena cava or the portal vein.
4. Combined form (20%).

6.10.9 Patent ductus arteriosus (PDA)

The ductus arteriosus represents a fetal communication between the left branch of the pulmonary artery and the aortic arch. This communication usually closes within the first month after birth. It can, however, remain patent (Fig. 6.74). PDAs are more common in premature babies, females, and in babies in whom there is a history of maternal rubella. The symptoms and signs related to the PDA depend on its size.

Small PDA

These are commonly asymptomatic and diagnosed at the time of routine medicals. A continuous, loud machinery murmur is heard infra-clavicularly on the left.

Large PDA

Infants with large PDAs may present with signs of congestive heart failure and the murmur may no longer be continuous due to the raised pulmonary artery pressure. The murmur is usually only heard in systole. The pulse may be collapsing and signs of left ventricular hypertrophy be detected. The ductus arteriosus is histologically composed of a media with spirally arranged smooth muscle fibres and a markedly thickened intima. Higher pressure in the aorta forces the arterial blood into the pulmonary circulation and thus overloads the right heart. PDAs may be complicated by heart failure, pulmonary hypertension, bacterial endocarditis and the development of Eisenmenger's syndrome.

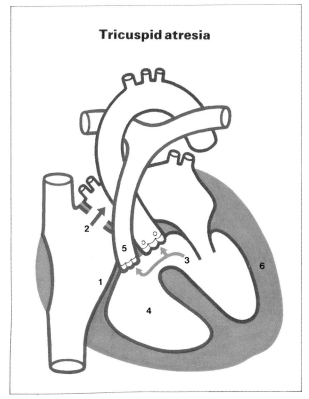

Fig. 6.77 Tricuspid atresia (1) with pulmonary artery hypoplasia (5), atrial (2) and ventricular septal defect (3), small right ventricle (4) and hypertrophy of left ventricular wall (6).

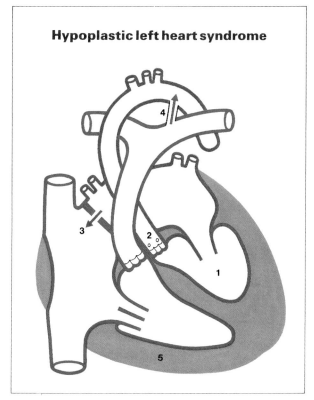

Fig. 6.78 Hypoplastic left heart syndrome. Small left ventricle (1), aortic hypoplasia (2), atrial septal defect (3), open ductus arteriosus (4), hypertrophy of the right ventricular wall (5).

6.10.10 Truncus arteriosus communis persistans

The following abnormalities are found:

1. Only one large artery with up to six semi-lunar valves (frequently four) arises from the heart.
2. The coronary arteries, pulmonary arteries and arteries of the head and upper limbs, as well as the descending aorta, will derive from the common vessel.
3. The pulmonary arteries may arise singly or from a common trunk.

The formation of a septum to separate the aorta and pulmonary trunk has not occurred developmentally. A common vessel overrides a VSD and transports mixed blood. Cyanosis is only slightly marked and is visible when the infant cries. With advancing age, the Eisenmenger reaction occurs and cyanosis increases.

6.10.11 Transposition of the great arteries

Transposition of the great arteries is characterized by the following developmental disorders:

1. The aorta arises from the right ventricle and transports venous blood and lies ventrally.
2. The pulmonary artery arises from the left ventricle, transports arterial blood and lies dorsally.

Transposition of the great arteries is the commonest cause of cyanotic heart disease in the newborn. Survival of the infant is dependent on the presence of a shunt to allow the blood from the two parallel circulations to mix.

Fallot's tetralogy

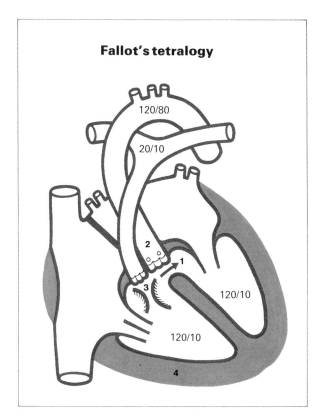

Fig. 6.79 Fallot's tetralogy with ventricular septal defect (1), central aorta (2), right infundibulum stenosis (3) and hypertrophy of the right ventricular wall (4).

Atrioventricular canal defect

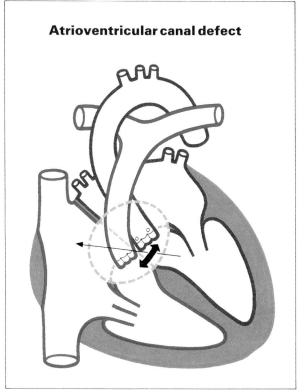

Fig. 6.80 Atrioventricular canal defect: defect of the lower atrial septum, abnormal connection between the left ventricle and right atrium (defect of valve flaps and septum).

6.10.12 Triscuspid atresia

Tricuspid atresia does not occur as an isolated defect but rather as part of a complex cardiac malformation. The blood flows from the right atrium to the left atrium via an ASD, then to the left ventricle. Part of the blood flows into the aorta and the rest of the blood goes through a VSD into the right ventricle, then to the pulmonary artery and the lungs. If the VSD is intact, the blood may pass through a PDA to the lungs. Clinically, cyanosis occurs immediately after birth and few children survive until the third year of life. The operative mortality for this condition is high with a 40% mortality.

6.10.13 Hypoplastic left heart syndrome

In this condition, left ventricular hypoplasia is found with atresia of the aorta, along with a paradoxical open foramen ovale, eccentric hypertrophy of the right heart and a patent PDA (Fig. 6.78). Mitral valve abnormalities and endocardial

fibrosis may also be present. The right ventricle takes over the cardiac function, the systemic circulation is fed through the PDA, so there is retrograde vascularization of the aortic arch and coronary arteries. The major clinical signs are hypotension and a blue-grey cyanosis. The mean life expectancy is two weeks.

6.10.14 Fallot's tetralogy

Fallot's tetralogy is the most common form of congenital cyanotic heart disease which presents after the first year of life (Fig. 6.79). This complex heart defect includes:

1. Pulmonary stenosis; this is infundibular or valvular in 75% of cases. The pulmonary artery is hypoplastic.
2. VSD.
3. Over-riding aorta.
4. Right ventricular hypertrophy.

If an ASD is also present, the condition is called Fallot's pentalogy. Children with Fallot's tetralogy

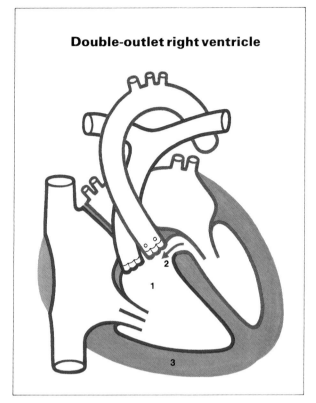

Double-outlet right ventricle

Fig. 6.81 **Double-outlet right ventricle:** Aorta and pulmonary artery spring from the common right ventricle (1) with hypertrophic wall (3), with ventricular septal defect (2) and small left ventricle.

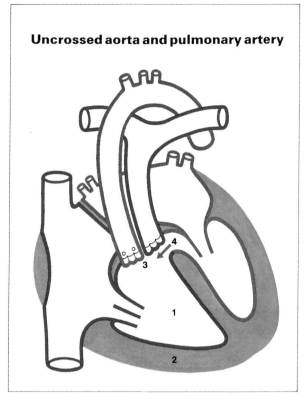

Uncrossed aorta and pulmonary artery

Fig. 6.82 **Uncrossed aorta and pulmonary artery** (3) arising from the right ventricle (1). Hypertrophy of the right ventricular wall (2) with high ventricular septal defect (4).

usually present in their first year of life with cyanotic attacks, which occur with crying or feeding. Dyspnoea, seizures and growth retardation are other presenting symptoms. The parents may describe that the child squats after mild exertion. This relieves the cyanosis by increasing the systemic resistance. Fallot's tetralogy may be complicated by cerebral abscesses, polycythaemia predisposing to arterial and venous thromboses, and bacterial endocarditis. The mean life expectancy is 12 years. On examination, a child with Fallot's tetralogy will be cyanosed, with a right ventricular heave, loud A2 and a loud ejection systolic murmur maximal in the pulmonary area.

6.10.15　Atrioventricular (AV) canal defects

The term AV canal defect refers to the various congenital cardiac defects of a particular region of

the heart, comprising the caudal part of the atrial septum, the AV valve and the cranial portion of the ventricular septum (Fig. 6.80). The defects are a result of incomplete growth of the AV endocardial cushions. The defects that can occur include the ASD primum type, cleft mitral and/or triscupid valve and a VSD.

6.10.16　Ebstein's anomaly

In this congenital disorder, the leaflets of the tricuspid valve are not attached in the correct positions. The anterior leaflet of the tricuspid valve is attached to the annulus. However, the other two leaflets are attached below the annulus on the right ventricular wall. This results in a large right atrium and small right ventricle. Ebstein's anomaly may be part of a complex cardiac malformation.

106

6.11 PERICARDIAL DISEASE

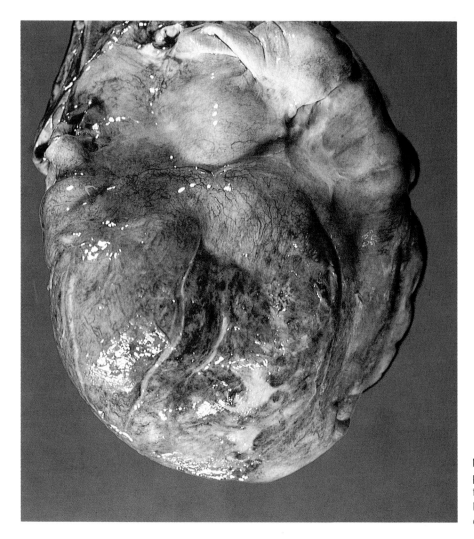

Fig. 6.83 Fibrinous pericarditis. Redness of the visceral pericardial layer and fibrin deposits over a myocardial infarct.

6.11.1 Pericardial effusion

Under physiological conditions the pericardial sac contains up to 150ml of a clear amber-coloured fluid. An increased amount of this serous fluid may be found in right heart failure and in conditions where there is hypoalbuminuria. A cholesterol-rich effusion may be found in rheumatoid arthritis or thyrotoxicosis. Blockage of the thoracic duct may lead to a chylous pericarditis. Coxsackie virus infection may lead to a recurrent benign pericarditis with an effusion. Haemorrhagic pericarditis may result from rupture of the left-to-right ventricle after myocardial infarction or after direct trauma such as bullet or stab wounds or after rupture of a dissecting aneurysm. Purulent effusion may be seen in cases of sepsis or as a result of an adjacent in-flammatory process (pneumonia, pleurisy or mediastinitis).

Clinical features

An effusion produces functional changes due to interference with diastolic filling which results in a rise in pressure in the pericardial cavity and the great vein. Pericardial tamponade may be the end result of pericardial effusion, and in haemorrhagic pericarditis may result when as little as 300ml of blood has been extravasated into the pericardium.

6.11.2 Pericarditis

This is the term for inflammation of the layers of the pericardium. It may be classified according to the

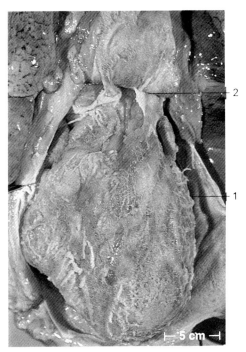

Fig. 6.84 Fibrinous pericarditis in uraemia.

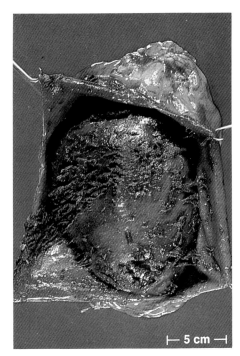

Fig. 6.85 Fibrinous-haemorrhagic pericarditis in tuberculosis.

cause of the inflammation (bacteria, viruses or occasionally parasites), or by toxic substances (uraemia), or by immunological processes (rheumatic pericarditis).

Fibrinous pericarditis

Both layers of the pericardium become coated with fibrin which forms long, grey-white villi as a result of contraction of the ventricles (Fig. 6.84). This is most commonly seen after myocardial infarction and in uraemia. It is usually suspected clinically by the finding of pericardial friction on auscultation. These sounds are transient and disappear rapidly as the effusion grows.

Haemorrhagic pericarditis

This is most commonly found after rupture of the left ventricular wall or in patients who have been over-anticoagulated. It may be rarely found in tuberculosis and following malignant involvement of the pericardium. It may present with pericardial pain, a friction rub on auscultation or with pericardial tamponade.

Fibrous or calcific pericarditis

The healing process of pericarditis may result in fibrous thickening of the pericardium and eventually calcification. The end-result is that the thickened pericardium restricts the normal heart movements and this may be a cause of long-term progressive heart failure.

6.12 HYPERTENSION

Hypertension is the chronic elevation of the arterial blood pressure above a normal value which is acceptable for the patient's age. With regard to the systolic blood pressure, this is usually accepted as 100 plus the chronological age of the patient and for the diastolic, it is usually above 90mmHg. Hypertension may be mainly systolic or may be a combination of systolic and diastolic. Systolic hypertension is particularly found in older people where the elasticity of the arterial tree has diminished significantly.

Incidence

The commonest form of hypertension is essential, i.e. no cause can be found for it. There may be a positive family history in up to one-third of the patients. A variety of other causes have been defined; in particular, renal hypertension may account for up to one-third of all cases of hypertension, with a small number of vascular and endocrine patients.

Risk factors

The risk factors are genetic, environmental, stress, neurogenic factors, obesity, metabolic disorders, hormonal and electrolyte imbalance.

6.12.1 Classification

In addition to the division of hypertension into primary and secondary according to aetiology, it may also be classified into benign and malignant forms according to the course it takes. The World Health Organization (WHO) divides hypertension into three categories.

I Primary (essential) hypertension
II Secondary hypertension

1. Renal hypertension
1.1 Hypertension resulting from renal parenchymatous disease

Acute and chronic glomerulonephritis
Chronic pyelonephritis
Polycystic kidneys
Systemic disease (diabetes mellitus, gout, amyloidosis and collagenosis)

1.2 Renovascular hypertension

Renal arterial stenosis
Renal artery occlusion
Renal artery aneurysm
Congenital and acquired arteriovenous fistula
Unusual conditions (renal cysts, hydronephrosis, compression due to tumours)

2. Cardiovascular causes
2.1 Increase in stroke volume

Total arteriovenous block
Aortic insufficiency
Arteriovenous fistulae
Patent ductus arteriosus
Anaemia
Polycythaemia rubra vera

2.2 Loss of elasticity of the aorta and great vessels
2.3 Aortic coarctation

3. Endocrine causes
3.1 Primary aldosteronism
3.2 Cushing's syndrome
3.3 Phaeochromocytoma
3.4 Drenogenital syndrome

4. Hypertension in hypercalcaemia
5. Hypertension in the new-born
6. Drug induced hypertension

	Main feature	Additional findings
Stage 1 (latent, labile hypertension) mild or borderline hypertension	High blood pressure 140–160mm Hg systolic 90–95mm Hg diastolic	Hyperkinetic circulation, heart rate and CO elevated. Vascular resistance normal, increased sympathetic activity, increased renin activity, fundus 0–1*
Stage 2 (fixed, stable hypertension) moderate hypertension	High blood pressure + left heart hypertrophy 160–180mm Hg systolic 95–115mm Hg diastolic	Normokinetic circulation, elevated systemic vascular resistance, fundus I–III
Stage 3 (advanced hypertension) severe hypertension	High blood pressure + left heart hypertrophy + organ damage over 180mm Hg systolic over 120mm Hg diastolic	Damage to heart, brain, kidneys; hypokinetic circulation at rest, reduced CO, greatly increased systemic vascular resistance, threatened heart failure, fundus II–IV

* Fundus	= optic fundus (increasingly severe modifications are meant)
Fundus 0–I	= no or only very slight optic fundus modifications
Fundus II	= arteriovenous nipping
Fundus III	= retinal haemorrhages
Fundus IV	= retinal haemorrhages and papilloedema

Fig. 6.86 Stages of hypertension.

6.12.2 Pathophysiology

The level of the arterial blood pressure results from a number of regulatory mechanisms which involve cardiac output, the central nervous system, adrenal gland and renal function. The relationship between cardiac output and peripheral resistance determines the blood pressure. However, both values can be influenced by the central nervous system via the sympathetic adrenal axis. In addition, the production of angiotensin and aldosterone plays a decisive role in the regulation of sodium and water excretion. Together with the dietary intake of salt and water, the secretion of these two substances determines the total fluid and sodium contents of the body, which in turn affects the blood volume and thus the ejection volume available. In addition to hereditary factors, stress and emotional upset may be associated with the development of high blood pressure by an action through the sympathetic adrenergic system. Such factors may be responsible for a rapid rise in blood pressure but it is doubtful if they are involved in sustained hypertension. In the early stages of hypertension, cardiac output is increased and peripheral resistance is reduced. It is not yet known if this is due to suppression of the baroreceptor reflex. In later, more advanced stages of hypertension, there is a rise in peripheral resistance due to an increase in tone of the resistive vessels and these in turn show increased reactivity due to the action of pressor substances such as angiotensin and noradrenaline. Whether the activation of the renin–angiotensin–aldosterone system plays a primary role in the development of hypertension remains unclear. It is known that sodium turnover is slowed down in patients with hypertension and that various tissues such as muscles, arteries and red cells in such patients have elevated intracellular sodium contents. By reducing the sodium intake, it is possible to bring the blood pressure of a number of hypertensive patients back into the normal range. Plasma renin activity is elevated in less than one-third of patients with hypertension and the role of this system in the aetiology of hypertension is unclear. It is also unknown if the observed elevation of plasma renin activity is the cause or consequence of high blood pressure. The extent to which the hypothetical natriuretic hormone and other possible pressor agents are responsible for hypertension remains unclear. In summary, the early stages of essential hypertension are characterized by a lability of blood pressure, by increased reactivity to external stimuli and it is unclear which of the various factors is most important.

6.12.3 Clinical examination

History

Patients with essential hypertension report symptoms that result from the effects of high blood pressure on the brain, heart, kidneys and peripheral vessels, i.e. exercise-induced breathlessness, palpitations, headaches, angina, depression and nose bleeds. In other family members of hypertensive patients, one should look for hypertension, obesity, stroke, premature heart attack, diabetes mellitus and gout. The patients should be asked about stress situations, dietary habits, in particular their salt intake, and current use of various medicines, such as analgesics and oral contraceptives.

Physical examination

Physical examination should be directed to the measurement of the blood pressure and the consequences of prolonged hypertension. Blood pressure should usually be measured after a period of rest with the patient seated, supine and then standing. The resting value gives a base line and the standing value shows the regulatory influence of the nervous and endocrine systems. Signs of left ventricular overload and decompensation must be looked for by auscultation of the heart and lungs. All pulses must be felt in order to detect the long-term sequelae of hypertension. Examination of the retina allows the severity and duration of hypertension to be graded.

Laboratory tests

These include the erythrocyte sedimentation rate, the red and white blood cell counts and haematocrit. The serum concentration of creatinine, urea, sodium, potassium, magnesium, bicarbonate, glucose, cholesterol, triglycerides and uric acid should also be estimated. Urine examination will give information on pH and the presence of glucose, protein or casts. A midstream sample of urine should be obtained for a qualitative and quantitative estimate of red cells, white cells and bacteria. These simple tests may give an early indication of the presence of endocrine disease or impairment of renal function.

ECG

The duration and severity of hypertension can also be estimated from the ECG, which may show left ventricular hypertrophy and strain, which may progress to left bundle branch block in the later stages. Episodes of atrial fibrillation, extrasystoles and other ventricular arrhythmias may also be observed in the ECG, particularly if coronary artery disease is present coincidentally.

Radiographic examination

X-ray of the chest should be taken first to determine heart size, to examine the shape of the left ventricle and the width of the aorta. Signs of left ventricular failure may also be found. An estimate of size of the kidneys may be made by an abdominal ultrasound, which may also show renal cysts, calcification or a renal tumour. Occasionally, tumours of the adrenal cortex may also be found on ultrasound but better images of both kidney and adrenal may be obtained with computer-assisted tomography, which may also diagnose abnormalities of the aorta. Special examinations: these include plasma hormone assays and measurement of plasma renin activity, endogenous catecholamines (adrenaline, noradrenaline), 24-hour urine excretion of vanilmandelic acid and the urinary catecholamines.

6.12.4 Types of hypertension

Primary hypertension

By primary or essential hypertension is meant any elevation of blood pressure which cannot be attributed to a detectable underlying pathology. It is the most common form of hypertension and is found in about 80% of hypertensive patients. It has a gradual onset, so that patients have few symptoms and these tend to arise later in the disease due to involvement of the heart, kidneys and cerebral vessels. Secondary hypertension results from disease of the kidneys, cardiovascular system, endocrine system or following certain types of therapy.

Mild hypertension

Mild hypertension is defined as a blood pressure which remains consistently above the upper limit of normal. The patient will have a diastolic blood pressure of between 90 and 105mmHg. Borderline hypertension is defined as a blood pressure between 105 and 120mmHg and severe hypertension above 120mmHg.

Malignant hypertension

In malignant hypertension or accelerated hypertension, there is usually marked elevation of the diastolic value above 120mmHg and this is associated with changes in blood vessels, especially in the retina, in which Grade IV changes are found. There are also lesions in the heart, kidneys and cerebral vessels and the patient is liable to have rapid onset of complications, such as cerebral haemorrhage, myocardial infarction or renal failure.

Hypertension in children

Hypertension may also be found in children. The borderline values are 110/70mmHg for children up to the age of six years, 120/75mmHg up to nine years and 130/80mmHg up to 14 years of age. Essential hypertension may be suspected if the blood pressure is persistently elevated in a child, when taken after an appropriate period of rest with the patient supine. Important factors to note are the presence of a family history and the presence of obesity. It has been estimated that between 1 and 12% of children and adolescents suffer from elevated blood pressure. Apart from essential hypertension in childhood, there are also secondary forms of hypertension caused by renal disease (polycystic kidney, renal hypoplasia, renal calcification due to idiopathic hypercalcaemia), cardiovascular diseases (coarctation, congenital arteriovenous valve formations), endocrine diseases (neuroblastoma) and diseases of the nervous system (cerebral haemorrhage due to birth trauma).

Hypertension in the elderly

Elevation of the blood pressure in excess of 180/100mmHg is often found in older patients (over the age of 65 years) and represents significant risk factors. Elderly patients are particularly liable to side-effects of antihypertensive therapy.

Hypertension in pregnancy

The blood pressure normally falls during pregnancy but between 5 and 15% of pregnant women exhibit an elevated blood pressure. This may represent previously undetected essential hypertension, undetected renal disease, or in the third trimester of pregnancy may represent pregnancy-induced hypertension. This latter may be associated with peripheral oedema, excess protein excretion in the urine and, if untreated, progress to eclampsia.

Renal hypertension

A distinction should be made between parenchymal disease of the kidneys as a cause of hypertension and renovascular causes. Parenchymal disease may be due to acute and chronic glomerulonephritis, pyelonephritis, polycystic kidney disease and systemic disorders affecting the kidney. The diagnosis may be suggested by the patient's symptoms (recurrent urinary tract infection or stone formation). Necrosis of the renal papillae, pyelonephritis or Kimmelstiel-Wilson's glomerulosclerosis may be observed in diabetes mellitus. Collagen disease (polyarteritis nodosa, lupus erythematosus) may also produce renal hypertension. In renovascular hypertension there is usually unilateral renal artery stenosis. Two forms of this may be found: the fibromuscular-dysplastic variety which involves the middle and distal third of the renal artery, and the atherosclerotic form which usually involves the origin of the renal artery at the aorta.

Cardiovascular hypertension

This is found in the following situations: increased stroke volume (in total AV block, aortic insufficiency, arteriovenous fistula, patent ductus arteriosus, anaemia), reduced elasticity of the aorta in the elderly and aortic coarctation.

Endocrine hypertension

Endocrine forms of hypertension are relatively rare and are usually due to disorders of the adrenal cortex or medulla. Such cases involve overproduction of adrenal cortical hormones, for example aldosterone in adrenal cortical adenoma (Conn's syndrome), cortisol in Cushing's syndrome, or noradrenaline, adrenaline and dopamine in tumours of the adrenal medulla. Systolic hypertension is also observed in hyperthyroidism as a result of the increased cardiac output.

Neurogenic hypertension

Hypertension may also be observed in diseases associated with increased intracranial pressure (head injury or cerebral damage due to chronic lead poisoning).

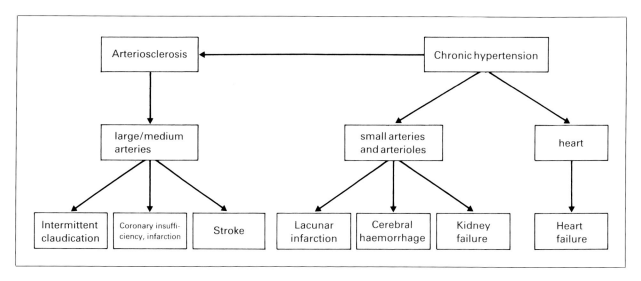

Fig. 6.87 Direct and indirect consequences of hypertension.

6.12.5 Complications

The effects of hypertension result from alteration of blood vessels in various organs, in particular, the kidneys, eyes, heart and brain.

Kidneys

In prolonged hypertension, degenerative arteriosclerosis or sclerotic changes develop in the kidneys, with thickening of the media associated with medial necrosis, loss of smooth muscle and atrophy of the glomeruli. These lesions rapidly result in renal impairment which is manifested by albuminuria, microhaematuria, impairment of renal function and a reduction in renal excretion of insulin and PAH clearance.

Eyes

Changes in the retinal blood vessels, which result in prolonged hypertension, include haemorrhages, exudates and oedema of the optic nerve head. These lead to impairment of vision and may result in blindness.

Heart

Prolonged hypertension may result in heart failure

or acute myocardial infarction and this is the cause of death in up to 70% of hypertensive patients.

Brain

The arteriosclerosis that results from prolonged hypertension leads to cerebral perfusion defects, cerebral haemorrhage and infarction. There may also be evidence of transient ischaemic attacks with unilateral paralysis, speech disturbance and focal seizures. A rapid rise in blood pressure may also produce hypertensive encephalopathy, the effects of which are probably due to cerebral oedema, and it manifests as severe headache, vomiting, visual disturbance, dizziness and epilepsy. Disorders of cerebral blood flow are the cause of death in about 16% of all hypertensive patients.

Definition

Hypotension is defined as a state in which the blood pressure falls below the lower normal limit (systolic 100mmHg and diastolic 60mmHg). Acute hypotension occurs in shock.

Classification

Chronic hypotension may be classified according to aetiology or to clinical criteria.

6.13 ARTERIAL HYPOTENSION

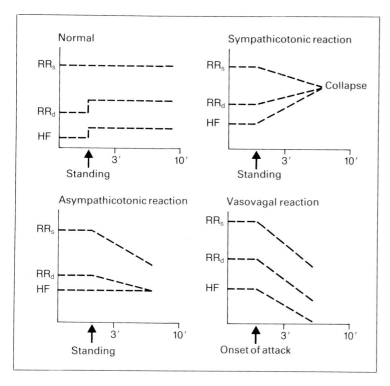

Fig. 6.88 Hypotension. Schellong test. Responses of the heart rate and the systolic and diastolic blood pressures.

Pathogenesis

There may be distinct entities; for example, primary or idiopathic hypotension is of unknown aetiology and secondary hypotension results from a variety of underlying disorders. These may include cardiac causes (heart failure, myocardial infarction, arrhythmias), hypovolaemia (bleeding, dehydration, burns), endocrine (adrenal, pituitary or thyroid insufficiency) or neurogenic (tabes dorsalis, syringomyelia, multiple sclerosis, alcoholism, diabetic neuropathy).

Iatrogenic hypotension is found after the administration of certain drugs (diuretics, vasodilators and anti-sympathetic drugs).

The clinical classification of hypotension can be considered in three sub-groups:

1. Asymptomatic chronic hypotension may be found in highly trained professional athletes.
2. Chronic hypotension, with clinical symptoms, may be found acutely or chronically.
3. Orthostatic hypotension may develop due to the sudden change in body position or after prolonged standing. Three forms may be distinguished:
   (i) Glycosympathetic tone, which may arise following prolonged bed rest, convalescence and in the absence of exercise. (ii) Positional hypotension, which occurs in elderly patients and also in patients with endocrine or neurological disease. (iii) Inappropriate vaso-vagal tone, where there is a sudden decrease in systolic or diastolic blood pressure as well as pulse rate and a syncopal attack may occur. The clinical picture is characterized by non-specific features. There may be constant fatigue, irritability, poor concentration, stabbing chest pains, buzzing in the ears and swimming vision. In extreme cases, there is a reduction of cerebral blood flow. The various forms of hypotension can be differentiated by measurement of pulse and blood pressure in various body positions.

6.13.1 Shock

The term shock means a state in which there is acute generalized peripheral circulatory failure resulting in a disturbance of tissue perfusion and cell damage. Shock leads to failure of various organs, for example, circulation, renal function and respiration. This is due to a fall in cardiac output. The

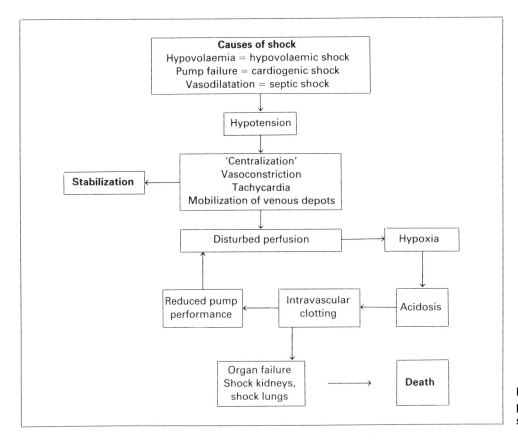

Fig. 6.89 Formal pathogenesis of shock.

speed at which cardiac output falls is of importance, as chronic diseases are tolerated better, for example, cardiac failure, cardiomyopathy.

Classification

The following types are recognized according to pathogenesis.

Hypovolaemic shock occurs if there is a decrease in the volume of circulating blood as a result of fluid or blood loss (for example after haemorrhage, burns or dehydration).

Cardiogenic shock results from pump failure after myocardial infarction, arrhythmias, myocarditis, acute valvular insufficiency or ineffective left ventricular filling. Reduced contractility of the ventricle is temporarily compensated by tachycardia and this is followed rapidly by a fall in cardiac output.

Septic shock (anaphylactic or neurogenic shock) is frequently found in cases of septicaemia due to Gram-negative organisms and may be attributed to a failure of peripheral circulatory regulation.

Pathogenesis and clinical features: shortly after the shock-inducing event, the blood pressure remains normal and the pulse rate is slightly increased. A fall in blood pressure is temporarily compensated by stimulation of baroreceptors and by the release of endogenous catecholamines. Peripheral resistance is increased by pre- and post-capillary vasoconstriction and venous return is enhanced by mobilization of venous pools. These effects are more noticeable in the skin, kidneys and splanchnic area, whereas the brain, heart and musculature retain their normal blood flow. In this phase, the patients are found to have a cold, pallid skin. As a result of the fall in perfusion, hypoxia and acidosis develop and, in some areas, statis of the circulation is evident, with aggregation of platelets and sludging of erythrocytes in the micro-circulation. Intravascular coagulation activation may also result. As perfusion deteriorates, a vicious circle is established, with pooling of blood in the micro-circulation followed by intravascular coagulation which leads to perfusion to organs continuing to diminish and consumption coagulopathy becoming more evident. The result of this is multi-organ failure, with rapid deterioration of renal function and respiratory insufficiency.

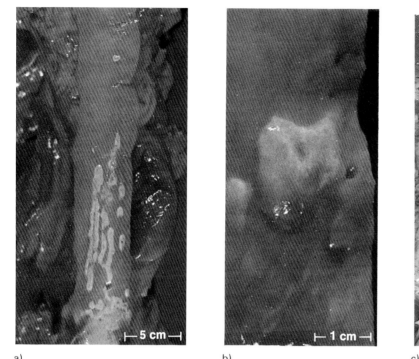
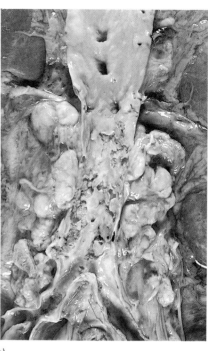

a)

b)

c)

Fig. 6.90 Aortic arteriosclerosis. a) and b) Lipid deposits, c) calcified arteriosclerosis with outgrowths.

6.14 ANGIOLOGY (ARTERIAL SYSTEM)

6.14.1 Arteriosclerosis

Definition

This is a general term for the ageing phenomenon of blood vessels in which there is an increase in fibrous tissue and a distinction has to be made between this ageing process and:

1. Atherosclerosis, which is defined by the WHO as a variable combination of changes of the intima of the arteries and it comprises a focal accumulation of lipids (Fig. 6.90), complex carbohydrates, blood and blood products, fibrous tissue and calcified deposits.
2. Non-specific internal fibrosis induced by an increase in blood pressure.
3. Monckeberg's medial sclerosis in which there is calcification of the media (goose-neck artery).
4. Genetic defects with vascular sclerosis.

Pathogenesis

Risk factors which promote the occurrence and development of arteriosclerosis are:

1. Age (over 40 years)
2. Sex (male)
3. Hypertension
4. Diabetes mellitus
5. Obesity/hyperlipoproteinaemia
6. Sedentary lifestyle
7. Cigarette smoking
8. Local haemodynamic vascular factors

Diabetes

Depending on the size of the blood vessels affected, macroangiopathy or microangiopathy may occur. In juvenile type I diabetes (i.e. insulin deficiency), microangiopathy develops first. In the case of maturity-onset type II diabetes (relative insulin deficiency), macroangiopathy is more prominent.

117

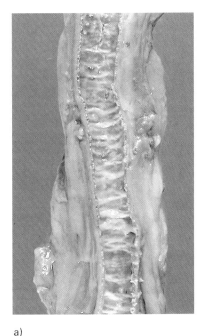
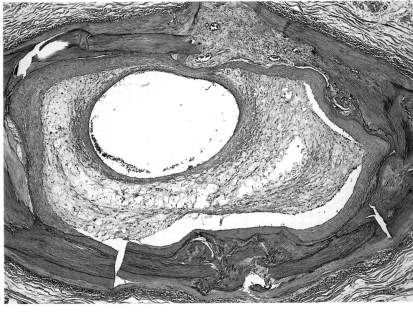

a)   b)

Fig. 6.91 Monckeberg's media calcification. a) 'String-of-pearls' artery. b) media calcification (blue spots in arterial wall) and intima fibrosis. HE stained.

During the prolonged course of diabetes, both forms of angiopathy merge with each other. The macroangiopathy is equivalent to arteriosclerosis and is associated with diabetes and hypertension. Microangiopathy can be detected by the PAS-positive thickening of the basal membranes in capillaries, arteries, arterioles and venules. In addition, there is proliferation of the intima similar to that found in endarteritis of small arteries and arterioles. Small aneurysms may also develop in the vessels of the brain and retina (diabetic retinopathy, which may progress to blindness). These, and similar lesions, are found in the renal glomeruli (Kimmelstiel-Wilson's glumerulosclerosis). Diabetic neuropathy is probably the result of angiopathy of the vasa nervorum.

Clinical features

This is a disease with a chronic progressive course which manifests itself after years by complications, which include local thrombosis or embolism lead-

ing to vascular occlusion with subsequent tissue ischaemia or as aneurysm which, on rupture, will produce clinical sequelae.

Pathology

Depending on the size of the vessels involved, various pathological changes result. These are particularly found in the aorta (an elastic artery) and include atheroma, calcification and hyaline change in smaller arterioles.

1. The gelatinous lesion which is found in the intima of the larger arteries is composed of fibres of collagen and intercellular deposits of glycosaminoglycans with lipids present in small amounts.
2. The lipid spot is composed of smooth muscle fibres, lipid-containing macrophages, necrotic cells and increased numbers of collagen fibres.
3. Fibrous plaques consist of increased numbers of muscle cells and collagen fibres. In addition, Sudan-positive material is deposited in variable

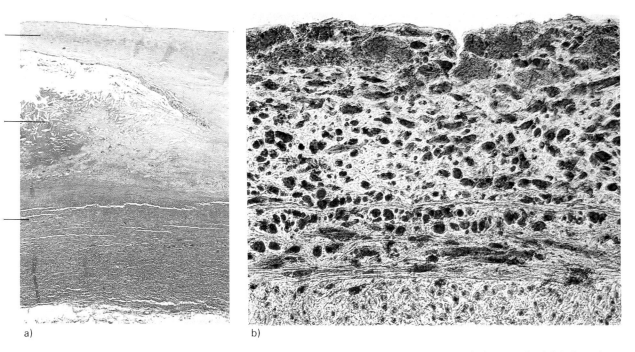

Fig. 6.92 Arteriosclerosis. a) Intima fibrosis with atheroma. HE stained. b) Sudan-stained atheroma bed, I: intima, A: atheroma, M: media.

amounts. Such fibrous plaques may be found before the age of 20 in the abdominal aorta and coronary arteries.

4. Atheroma consists of a central necrotic and often ulcerated fibrous plaque which may contain amounts of calcium and cholesterol crystals. There may be atrophy of the media under the atheromatous plaque and the adventitia contains inflammatory exudates. The characteristic complications of atheroma include classification, thrombosis on its surface, obstruction of blood flow and aneurysm formation due to weakening of the vessel wall. Emboli consisting of fibrin platelet material or lipid-rich constituents of the atheromatous plaque may also be present.

6.14.2 Fibromuscular dysplasia

This is an idiopathic segmental stenosis of a muscular artery (e.g. renal artery) and is not due to atheroma or inflammatory infiltration. Women are affected five times more frequently than men and fibromuscular dysplasia may account for up to 20% of hypertension in which both renal arteries may be affected as well as individual branches. The obstruction may be focal (up to 1cm long) or tubular (over 1cm long) and, on angiography, gives the appearance of multiple lesions (string-of-pearls variant). Histologically, the media is more commonly affected (80% of cases). In the other 20% of cases, the fibromuscular dysplasia affects the intima with concentric fibrosis.

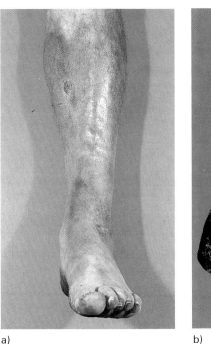 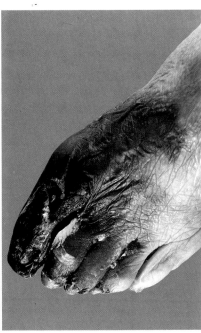 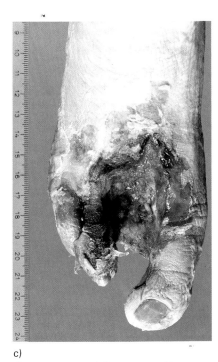

a) b) c)

Fig. 6.93 Occlusive arterial disease. a) Skin necrosis with demarcation. b) Extensive gangrene. c) Gangrene with partial slough.

6.14.3 Occlusive arterial disease

The most common underlying disorder in occlusive arterial disease (OAD) is arteriosclerosis plus or minus the presence of embolism or thrombosis (Fig. 6.93). Other vascular causes are much rarer and include obliterative thromboangiitis, polyarteritis nodosa, etc. There may be a background of diabetes mellitus.

Causes

1. Arterial embolism is found in 70% of cases, mainly originating from the heart (either valves or mural thrombosis following myocardial infarction). Aortic aneurysm may also be present.
2. In up to 20% of cases, local thrombosis may be the cause.
3. In under 10% of cases, dissecting aneurysm or local vascular trauma may be found.

Clinical features

The clinical symptoms of occlusive arterial disease include calf pain on walking (intermittent claudication) and there may be episodes of acute sudden onset pain indicating an acute arterial occlusion. The walking distance of the patient becomes progressively less as the disease progresses. The distribution of the pain gives a clue as to which vessels are obstructed. As time goes on, there may be pain occurring particularly at night time, which is not associated necessarily with exertion. Eventually, trophic changes occur in the skin and this may rapidly progress to gangrene. This is a disease of the elderly and is found more commonly in men, with a sex ratio of 4 : 1. Approximately 30% of patients have a history of diabetes mellitus.

Occlusive arterial disease may be staged by the method of Fontaine-Ratschow.

Stage I: Symptoms occur during extreme effort. The extent of the disease may be found by angiography.

Stage II: Symptoms after physical exertion. There is reduced exercise tolerance (intermittent claudication). A sub-classification of stage IIa and IIb may be used. In IIa the distance that can be walked is still adequate for normal lifestyle, but in stage IIb the patient is unable to work because of the onset of calf pain.

Stage III: There is pain at rest due to the failure of the collateral circulation and, indeed, pain may be induced when the limb is raised then lowered. Objective testing shows defective circulation to the periphery.

Stage IV: Trophic changes become well advanced and may proceed to gangrene. The clinic-

120

al diagnosis is supported by various functional tests (positional tests: fist test, Allan test, Adson test and walking test), as well as non-invasive and invasive procedures, such as oscillography, rheography, ultrasound Doppler, thermography and arteriography.

Localization of the vascular occlusion may be possible by the positioning of the pain:

Pain	*Occluded vessel*
Foot	Femoral arteries
Calf	Above the popliteal artery
Thigh	Above the groin
Buttocks	Aorta to the internal iliac artery

This provides a classification of occlusive arterial disease to include:

1. Peripheral disease of the arms and legs
2. Upper limb type with femoro-popliteal occlusion
3. Pelvic type with aorto-iliac occlusion
4. Pectoral girdle type with aortic arch, carotid artery and subclavian variety
5. Organ occlusion (renal artery, mesenteric artery, etc.)

6.14.4 Aortic arch syndrome

In this syndrome there is narrowing of the arteries of the head and upper limbs (brachio-cephalic trunk, subclavian and carotid). A collateral circulation may develop only when the occlusion is located close to the aorta. The clinical features depend on the position of the occlusion and its duration, for example, carotid occlusion may give rise to basilar insufficiency and subclavian occlusion to pain in the upper limbs. Vertebral steal syndrome (subclavian steal syndrome): in some cases of occlusion of the subclavian artery, a reversed circulation of the blood may occur. The upper limbs are then supplied by the vertebral artery with the result that cerebral circulation is reduced. A similar situation may also occur with carotid occlusion, in which case the reverse circulation is through the internal carotid artery to the external carotid artery.

6.14.5 Mesenteric arterial stenosis

Narrowing of the mesenteric artery may lead to colicky pain after eating (abdominal angina). Com-

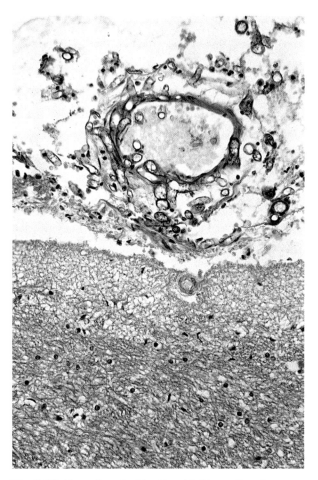

Fig. 6.94 Mycotic arteritis. Fungi in the wall and surroundings of a meningeal vessel. Brain tissue at the bottom of the picture. Grocot stained.

plete occlusion leads to mesenteric infarction. The clinical stages include:

1. An initial stage of up to 6 hours, which is characterized by abdominal pain and diarrhoea. Signs of shock may rapidly develop.
2. The silent interval between 7 and 12 hours, which is characterized by continuous pain, a rapid deterioration in the clinical condition of the patient with absent intestinal peristalsis, and it is probable that irreversible ischaemia of the bowel has now occurred.
3. The terminal stage, over 12 hours, in which the patient presents with paralytic ileus and the features of peritonitis and shock.

6.14.6 Renal artery stenosis

The commonest variety of this is in the elderly, in which there is severe arteriosclerosis. In younger

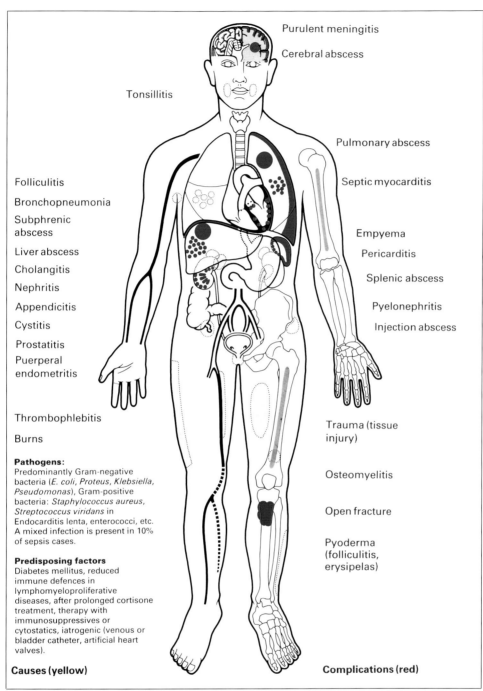

Purulent meningitis

Cerebral abscess

Tonsillitis

Pulmonary abscess

Septic myocarditis

Folliculitis

Bronchopneumonia

Subphrenic abscess

Liver abscess

Cholangitis

Nephritis

Appendicitis

Cystitis

Prostatitis

Puerperal endometritis

Empyema

Pericarditis

Splenic abscess

Pyelonephritis

Injection abscess

Thrombophlebitis

Burns

Trauma (tissue injury)

Osteomyelitis

Open fracture

Pyoderma (folliculitis, erysipelas)

Pathogens:
Predominantly Gram-negative bacteria (*E. coli*, *Proteus*, *Klebsiella*, *Pseudomonas*), Gram-positive bacteria: *Staphylococcus aureus*, *Streptococcus viridans* in Endocarditis lenta, enterococci, etc. A mixed infection is present in 10% of sepsis cases.

Predisposing factors
Diabetes mellitus, reduced immune defences in lymphomyeloproliferative diseases, after prolonged cortisone treatment, therapy with immunosuppressives or cytostatics, iatrogenic (venous or bladder catheter, artificial heart valves).

Causes (yellow)

Complications (red)

Fig. 6.95 Metastatic sepsis.

patients the causation is fibromuscular dysplasia. Progressive reduction in renal blood flow leads to hypertension (up to 25% of all causes of hypertension). Clinically, there is an elevated diastolic blood pressure in young patients and this may be confirmed by arteriography.

6.15 ANGIITIS

This is an inflammation of the blood vessels or lymphatics.

Classification

Vascular inflammation (angiitis) may be found in the arteries (arteritis), capillaries (capillaritis), veins (phlebitis), or lymph vessels (lymphangiitis). The entire vascular wall may be affected (panangiitis), or only part of it (for example, endangiitis, mesaortitis, periarteritis). If the inflammatory process starts in the vessel and then extends into the surrounding tissues, this may be called primary angiitis. If the inflammatory process involves the

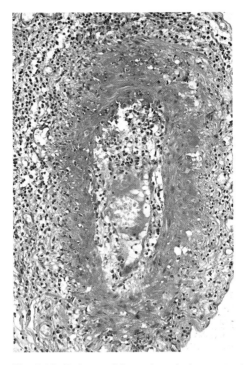

Fig. 6.96 Polyarteritis nodosa in the acute stage. HE stained.

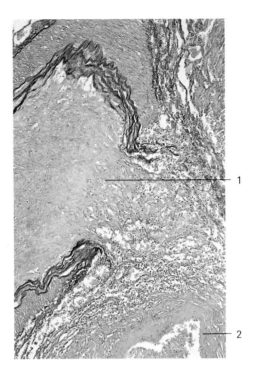

Fig. 6.97 Polyarteritis nodosa with scarring and with partial disruption of the vessel wall by granulation tissue. Van Gieson stained. 1: Wall defect. 2: Fresh fibrinoid necrosis.

vessel only as part of a local inflammatory reaction, this may be called secondary angiitis. The other name is concomitant angiitis, for example, if the inflammation extends from local ulceration, tumours and a range of other disorders. Angiitis may be caused by a range of pathogenic processes, physical or chemical.

6.15.1 Virus angiitis

In some viral disorders, there is a selective injury to the endothelium, so that the haemorrhagic component dominates the histological picture (influenza and measles).

6.15.2 Angiitis caused by *Rickettsia*, *Chlamydia* and *Treponema*

Rickettsia and *Chlamydia* are selectively localized to the reticulo-endothelial system (RES). There may also be selective involvement of cutaneous blood vessels. In the case of tertiary syphilis the vasa vasorum are primarily affected and this leads to alteration of the aortic media (mesaortitis) and also changes in smaller arteries of the brain.

6.15.3 Bacterial angiitis

This is a severe inflammation of the small arteries and capillaries and is observed in septicaemia caused by Gram-positive or Gram-negative bacteria. The foci of infection tend to be in the renal glomerular, myocardial and pulmonary capillaries. It may also be found in the umbilical vein (omphalophlebitis), in which case the infection arises from the area of the intrahepatic portal vein (peylophlebitis). In addition, angiitic changes may be a manifestation of allergy to bacteria.

6.15.4 Parasitic angiitis

Various parasites may multiply and spread long blood and lymph vessels and cause changes by their very presence (schistosomiasis, filariasis, onchocercosis).

6.15.5 Mycotic angiitis

Fungal disorders may also affect the vascular system, for example candidiasis. Among the nonspecific causes of vascular inflammation is the effect

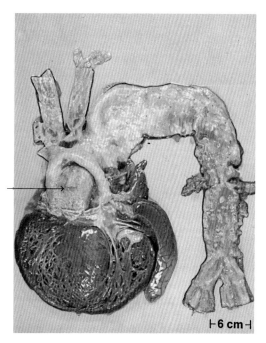

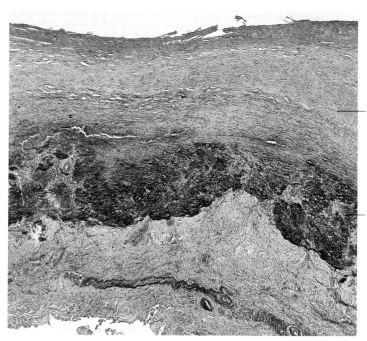

Fig. 6.98 Syphilitic mesaortitis. Dilatation of the thoracic aorta and aneurysm in the descending aorta (→).

Fig. 6.99 Syphilitic mesaortitis. Breakdown of the media (1) with intima fibrosis (2). Elastica-nuclear true red stained.

of ionizing radiation, which causes endothelial loss acutely and which may later lead to fibrosis and vascular occlusion. Vascular injury may also be caused by heat and cold, as well as chemical agents, for example, intravenous injection of drugs.

6.15.6 Septicaemia

The effects of septicaemia may be local or generalized and may affect the lymphatic system as well as the blood vessels. The presence of pathogenic bacteria in the blood (sepsis) is usually associated with dramatic clinical signs. The clinical symptoms are rigors, shivering and fever. The diagnosis is confirmed by finding the pathogenic bacteria, usually from repeated blood cultures. Shock may result, especially in the case of a Gram-negative septicaemia.

6.15.7 Polyarteritis nodosa (pan- or periarteritis)

In this, there may be segmental, necrotic, immunologically regulated inflammation of the medium-sized and small arteries, associated with vascular occlusion and infarction of tissue (Fig. 6.96). Men are particularly involved in the middle years of life.

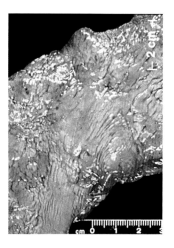

Fig. 6.100 Intimal scars in syphilitic mesaortitis.

Pathogenesis

This is unknown but it is thought that it may have an immunological basis.

Pathology

The small arteries of the kidneys, heart and liver, gastro-intestinal tract, testes, skin and CNS are most frequently affected. In addition, large lymph nodes are occasionally seen along the course of the

124

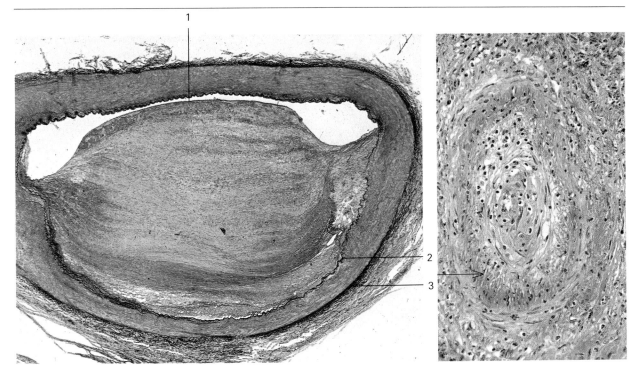

Fig. 6.101 Obliterative endangiitis. Narrowing of the lumen by cushion-shaped intimal thickening. Elastica-nuclear true red stained. 1: intimal thickening. 2: internal elastic lamina. 3: external elastic lamina.

Fig. 6.102 Reactive obliterative endangiitis in the base of a peptic ulcer. HE stained. (→ media).

vessels and four stages are recognized histologically:

1. Fibrinoid necrosis stage: both intima and media are affected segmentally. There is fibrinoid necrosis with degeneration of the elastic internal lamina. This is determined by staining homogeneously with eosin and Van Gieson. There may also be associated thrombosis on the endothelium.
2. Cellular reaction stage: the entire vascular wall, including the adventitia, is densely infiltrated with cells. Usually these are neutrophil granulocytes, lymphocytes, plasma cells and histiocytes. Eosinophilic granulocytes may also be seen. The segmental nature of the disease is still present at this stage.
3. Granulomatous reaction stage: proliferation of the intimal cells leads to intimal thickening with obstruction of the lumen. After the internal elastic lamina has broken down, micro-aneurysms form.
4. Scarring stage: after regression of the inflammatory exudate, there is formation of fibrous scars. The associated veins are largely unaffected in all these phases.

Clinical features

The clinical presentation depends on the organs affected. This may often be very difficult as the vascular changes occur sequentially. The diagnosis is confirmed by histological means, for example needle biopsy of the kidney. The prognosis is dependent on the time at which treatment is started.

6.15.8 Vascular disease

Vascular disease is a common feature of syphilis due to the presence of *Treponema pallidum*. In the tertiary stages, there are usually changes in the aorta and in the medium-sized cerebral arteries.

Syphilitic mesaortitis (Figs 6.98–6.100) is a typical complication of tertiary syphilis and occurs mainly in the elderly. The ascending aorta is usually affected macroscopically with dilatation and perhaps aneurysm formation. The aortic valve cusps may also be affected and become roughened and this inflammatory reaction may narrow the ostia of the coronary arteries. Histologically, the disease process starts with a lymphocytic infiltration in the vaso vasorum. The small vessels show endarteritis and this produces a failure of nutritional flow to the aortic wall. The medial necrosis starts with degeneration of elastic fibres which are replaced by collagen. This, in turn, leads to marked thinning of the vessel wall and loss of elasticity.

The small arteries at the base of the brain and in the hemispheres become infiltrated with plasma

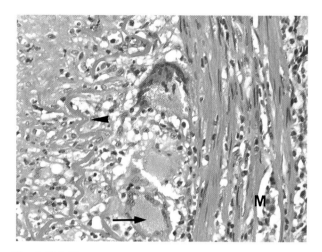

Fig. 6.103 Temporal arteritis with foreign-body giant cells (→). HE stained.
◀ : elastica interna. M: media.

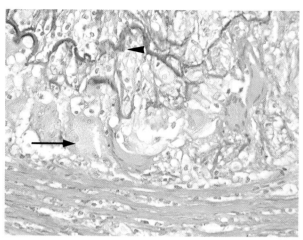

Fig. 6.104 Temporal arteritis. Splitting and breakdown of elastic fibres and the presence of multinuclear giant cells (→). Elastica van Gieson stained.
◀ : elastica interna.

cells and small gummae may form (Baumgarten's syphilitic periarteritis or Hubener's syphilitic end-arteritis).

Clinical features

The narrowing of the coronary arteries leads to myocardial ischaemia and this is exacerbated by the distortion of the aortic valve cusps, which produces aortic insufficiency and hence a reduction in diastolic filling of the coronary arteries. Later features of the intrathoracic aortic aneurysm supervene.

6.15.9   Obliterative angiitis (thromboangiitis obliterans, Winnie Waterburger disease)

This may be defined as a segmental inflammation of medium-sized arteries and veins, characterized by intimal fibrosis and thrombosis. The lower limbs of young men are usually affected but other organs may also be affected (heart, brain, gastrointestinal tract). (See Figs 6.101, 6.102.)

Pathogenesis

Genetic factors have been implicated; for example there is an increased incidence in the Far East and also in Israel. In the western world, the most important exogenous factor is cigarette smoking.

Pathology

Microscopically, the vessels appear greatly narrowed and the following features may be diagnosed histologically.

1. Acute phase: diffuse inflammatory infiltration with lymphocytes, plasma cells and occasional granulocytes are found in all layers of the vessel wall and their presence may be associated with the onset of local thrombosis which is rapidly organized. The internal elastic lamina remains intact.
2. The subacute phase: here, there are circumscribed medial necrotic lesions with occasional giant cells of a foreign body type.
3. The chronic phase: here, organization of thrombi is prominent, with the result that the intima becomes thickened and obstruction of arterial flow occurs. The clinical features are those of disturbance of blood flow, usually starting with intermittent claudication and followed by the onset of gangrene of the extremities. There may also be infarction of the internal organs.

6.15.10   Concomitant fibrous arteritis

There may be intimal fibrosis with narrowing and obliteration of the vessel lumen. This may be found in situations adjacent to chronic peptic ulceration.

6.15.11   Temporal arteritis (Figs 6.103, 6.104)

This is a systemic giant cell arteritis in which there is involvement of the medium and larger elastic muscular arteries. This is particularly seen in the temporal artery and its branches and the branches of the carotid artery. It has a predilection for women in later years (70–75).

Pathogenesis

The pathogenesis of the disease is uncertain. It has been suggested that there may be an auto-immune element as over 70% of patients with temporal arteritis also have polymyalgia rheumatica with involvement of the muscles of the shoulder girdle or occasionally the pelvic girdle.

Pathology

The temporal artery may be palpated due to its extreme thickening. Histologically, three stages may be differentiated. In the initial phase, the intima is thickened by the presence of a fibrinous cellular reaction. The result is the loss of the vessel lumen and also loss of the internal elastic lamina. In the later phase, the histological picture is dominated by a granulomatous reaction with giant cells of a foreign body type which appear to phagocytose the internal elastic lamina. There may be local thrombotic events and tissue necrosis. In the later phases, severe scarring and distortion of the vessel wall occur and there is progressive fibrosis with progressive loss of blood flow.

Clinical features

The clinical picture is characterized by loss of appetite, headache, an elevated erythrocyte sedimentation rate and high levels of gamma globulin. There is an association with acute onset of stroke and if the ophthalmic artery is involved, as it is in 60% of cases, blindness is an important complication. The diagnosis is established by histological study of a temporal artery segment at biopsy. Treatment is with early high dose corticosteroids.

OTHER FORMS OF VASCULITIS

6.15.12   Allergic vasculitis with granuloma formation (Churg-Strauss disease)

This is a disease with the changes similar to those found in polyarteritis nodosa but with simultaneous involvement of the accompanying veins and also the pulmonary arteries. In addition, there is peripheral eosinophilia in the blood and in the tissues. Small foci of epithelioid cells, with or without central fibrinoid necrosis, are also found. The finding of polyarteritis nodosa with eosinophilia and signs of bronchial asthma is also of clinical relevance. There is an overlap between polyarteritis nodosa and Churg-Strauss disease.

6.15.13   Hypersensitivity vasculitis (allergic vasculitis, anaphylactoid purpura)

This is an inflammatory process of the cutaneous venules (capillaries and arterioles may also be involved). There is leucocytic infiltration with migration of leucocytes through the vascular wall. The following are associated pathological processes (ulcerative colitis, chronic active hepatitis, primary biliary cirrhosis), collagenoses (systemic lupus erythematosus, rheumatoid arthritis), Henoch-Schoenlein purpura, viral or bacterial infectious diseases, serum sickness and reactions to medicines such as antibiotics, sulphonamides and cytostatics.

The dominant clinical findings are papular or purpuric-like skin changes. The diagnosis is confirmed by skin biopsy and the finding of the typical histological picture.

6.15.14   Wegener's granulomatosis

This is a necrotic granulomatous vasculitis involving the upper respiratory tract, lungs and kidneys. The disease occurs more frequently in men than women and the mean age of the patients is 40–50 years.

Pathogenesis

The cause is unknown. It has been postulated that an immune basis may be present.

Pathology

Macroscopically, the nasal mucosa appears to be ulcerated and rounded areas of necrosis are found in the lungs. Necrotic and granulomatous changes are found histologically adjacent to small arteries and veins. The lesions are characterized by fibrinoid necrosis, epithelioid cell nodules and multinuclear giant cells. These changes are found both in the vascular wall and in the surrounding tissues.

Clinical features

Wegener's granulomatosis must be differentiated from the fatal mid-line syndrome. This is an inflammatory disease of the airways but without involvement of the kidney. In addition, there is a very rare lymphomatoid granulomatosis which has been described predominantly in young women. In this, there is a lymphocytic plasma cell infiltration of pulmonary vessels with necrosis and destruction of the vascular wall.

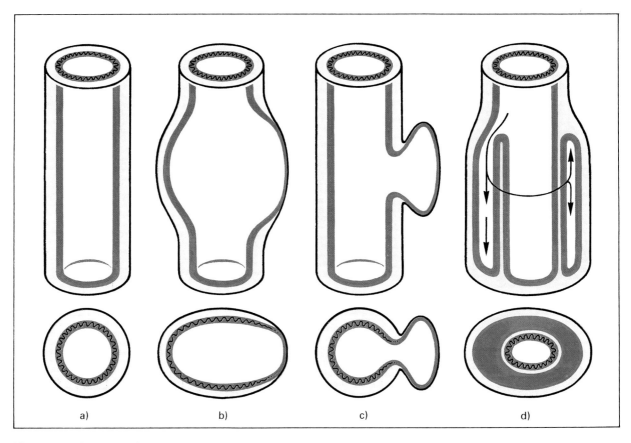

Fig. 6.105 Diagram of forms of aneurysm.
a) Normal. b) Fusiform. c) Saccular. d) Dissecting.

6.15.15   Mucocutaneous lymph node syndrome (Kawasaki's disease)

This is a condition usually observed in children and young adolescents in Japan. It consists of swelling of the cervical lymph nodes and angiitis. This resembles polyarteritis nodosa, with particular involvement of the coronary arteries. The cause is unknown.

6.15.16   Takayasu's arteritis (idiopathic aortitis, aortic arch syndrome)

This is a disease of unknown aetiology usually affecting young women. The changes occur usually in the large elastic arteries (aortic arch, descending aorta, major organ and limb arteries). Histologically, there is granulomatous infiltration and fibrosis. The clinical manifestations depend almost totally on the vascular segment involved.

6.16   ANEURYSMS

Definition

These are circumscribed, congenital or acquired pathological dilatations of the arterial lumen or heart wall.

Incidence

Aneurysms are common in the aorta (Fig. 6.105). Dissecting aneurysm and syphilitic aneurysm occur mainly in the ascending aorta. Atherosclerotic ones (Fig. 6.106) are usually found in the arch and descending aorta and some of the smaller arteries of the limbs (popliteal artery) and organs (basilar artery of the brain, renal artery, splenic artery). Aneurysms are rarely observed in the pulmonary vessels. Men are affected more often than women with a sex ratio of 2 : 1 (women may have aneurysms of the basilar artery twice as often as men). Aneurysms occur in the older age groups and peak between 50–70 years.

Pathogenesis

Aneurysms may be congenital or acquired. In the circle of Willis, they are usually single. Dissecting aneurysms may be found associated with certain congenital diseases, such as Marfan's syndrome, Ehlers-Danlos syndrome and pseudoxanthoma elasticum – Darier's disease). Among the causes of acquired aneurysm are hypertension, aortic medial necrosis, Erdheim-Gsell's disease 10%, syphilis 5%, trauma 1% and other factors, such as infection or inflammation.

Pathology

It is important to make a distinction between a true aneurysm, which affects all layers of the vascular wall, and of false aneurysm, which may develop after intimal injury. In this situation, blood infiltrates the vascular wall and is contained only by the thickened adventitia or inflammatory response. This process corresponds to a wall haematoma. The following types of aneurysm may be distinguished with regard to their morphology and extent.

Saccular aneurysms are spherical with a small connecting pathway to the blood vessel and they have defined boundaries.

Fusiform aneurysms are spindle-shaped aneurysms which occur on one side of the vessel, or alternatively, they may affect the entire circumference of the vessel. The boundaries are not defined.

Dissecting aneurysms result from a tear in the intima, the blood infiltrating the vessel wall between the intima and the adventitia. There are various other unusual forms, for example, the tortuous aneurysm. This is a dilated artery running in a series of loops (mostly found in the splenic artery). Several arterial branches are affected. A cirsoid aneurysm is present. The term mycotic aneurysm designates a dilatation of the vascular wall caused by inflammation, for example as a result of bacterial endocarditis. An arteriovenous aneurysm results from the presence of an arteriovenous fistula.

Histology

The histological changes depend on the causation of the aneurysm. In general, there is thinning of the media with degeneration and splitting of the elastic fibres and replacement with collagen. There may be overlying thrombi found in the lumen of the associated vessels.

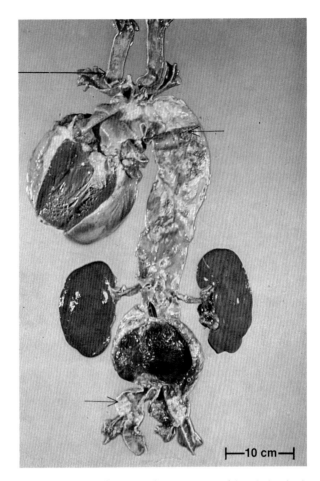

Fig. 6.106 Arteriosclerotic aneurysm of the abdominal aorta. Upper arrow = cervical vessel. Centre arrow = descending aorta. Lower arrow = common iliac artery.

Clinical features

Aneurysms may have a chronic and largely asymptomatic clinical course. Only about 20% of aneurysms are detected before autopsy. Large aneurysms may be found on routine palpation or may present with disorders of blood flow or rupture. Leaking of an abdominal aortic aneurysm produces the features of retroperitoneal haemorrhage and the diagnosis is confirmed by CT or ultrasound.

6.17 INTRAMURAL HAEMATOMA

This is a localized haematoma within the wall of the artery and usually results from local trauma. The intima usually remains intact and there is no thrombus formation over it.

129

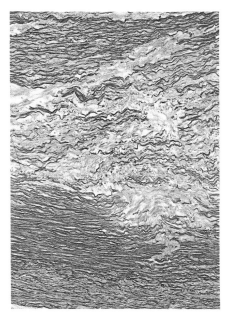

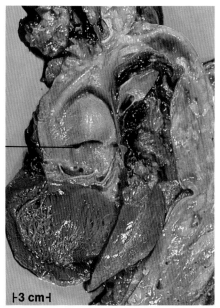

|-3 cm-|

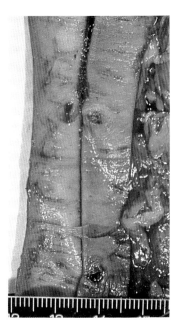

Fig. 6.107 Medial necrosis with lake-like mucopolysaccharide deposits in the media. Elastica van Gieson stained.

Fig. 6.108 Dissecting aneurysm: Lateral tear in the ascending aorta (arrow).

Fig. 6.109 Dissecting aneurysm: Walls of the aorta displayed.

6.18 ARTERIOVENOUS FISTULA

Arteriovenous fistulae are abnormal communications between arteries and veins. They may be congenital or acquired. The acquired variance may result from local trauma, inflammation, erosion or may be produced by surgery. Congenital arteriovenous fistulae may be associated with enlargement of the limb (haemangiectatic hypertrophy, Klippel-Trenaunay syndrome, Parkes-Weber syndrome). There may be local disturbance of blood flow with an increased venous return and local venous dilatation and this, in turn, may lead to necrosis and bleeding. With very large arteriovenous malformations, there may be an increased cardiac output and the possibility of long-term heart failure.

Klippel-Trenaunay syndrome is due to a congenital arteriovenous malformation and the manifestations start in early childhood with partial giantism, accompanied by the obvious vascular defect. There is usually enlargement of the affected limb. Parkes-Weber syndrome may also be associated with arteriovenous fistula formation.

6.19 ERDHEIM-GSELL'S MEDIAL NECROSIS AND DISSECTING ANEURYSM

6.19.1 Erdheim-Gsell's medial necrosis

This is an idiopathic cystic medial necrosis in which there is degeneration of the elastic fibres and the smooth muscle of the aortic media and there are associated deposits of an acid mucopolysaccharide. These deposits are alcian positive and PAS negative. Increased deposition of fibrous tissue is shown on Van Gieson staining, which shows yellow, homogeneous deposits in the media. The cause of this disease is unknown and all age groups and both sexes are affected. The mean age of diagnosis is 50 years.

6.19.2 Dissecting aneurysm

As a result of a tear of the intima, blood infiltrates the arterial wall (usually the aorta). A blunt chest trauma may be the initial cause of the tear in a few cases but usually there is no history of injury prior to the event. In a small number of cases there may be a defect of the aortic wall, for example Marfan's syndrome, Ehlers-Danlos syndrome or medial necrosis.

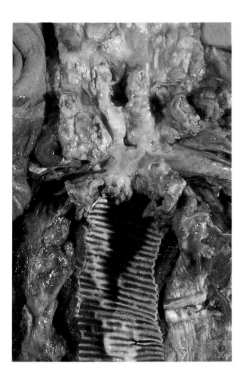

Fig. 6.110 Aortic replacement by prosthesis.

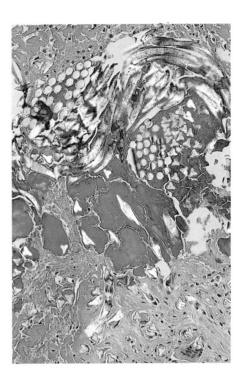

Fig. 6.111 Foreign body reaction involving giant cells in response to the prosthetic material (double-refraction in polarized light). HE stained, POL.

Pathology

The aorta shows a transverse tear often just above the aortic valve. The blood spreads within the wall between the intima and the media and dissects the vascular layers. If the dissection is extensive, other blood vessels may be involved, for example the renal arteries, and the dissection may extend as far as the pelvic vessels to form a pelvic haematoma. There may be reperforation and re-entry into the lumen of the aorta further down, in which case spontaneous healing can occur, although this is rare. The usual result is external perforation into the mediastinum, retroperitoneal tissues or pericardium. The result is catastrophic bleeding. Clinically, the first event may be manifested as acute pain often between the shoulder blades. The diagnosis is best confirmed by oesophageal ultrasound or computer-assisted tomography.

6.20 VESSEL REPLACEMENT

In occlusive arterial disease, an organ or limb may be salvaged by replacing the stenosed arterial segment. A variety of materials may be used for vessel grafts, for example (a) vessels from other parts of the patient's own body, usually veins. These are of value in grafting small and medium-sized arteries but are of little value in larger vessels. (b) Arteries removed at autopsy and lyophilized and stored have been used. These are not very satisfactory as they usually always calcify when transplanted into other patients. (c) A range of artificial materials have also been used to form vascular grafts, in particular fine-meshed poly-tetrafluoroethylene (PTFE) and dacron (Fig. 6.110). After implantation, the grafts usually become coated with fibrin and some of this may be endothelialized. In some patients there may be an inflammatory reaction to the presence of the artificial material and this can result later in thrombotic occlusion.

6.21 FUNCTIONAL BLOOD FLOW DISORDERS

Under this heading are included a variety of arterial disorders in which the aetiology is not understood.

6.21.1 Raynaud's disease

Definition

This is an intermittent, occlusive disorder of the digital arteries, usually resulting from exposure to cold in which there are a series of changes in the skin, with the triphasic colour change red to blue to white. It is a disease mainly of women (80%) and occurs after puberty. The patient frequently complains of migraine.

Pathogenesis

The pathogenesis of this condition is unknown. It has been suggested that there may be increased sympathetic tone. It is only in patients with secondary Raynaud's syndrome that an associated pathology may be found, such as trauma due to vibration (pneumatic drill disease), cold agglutination disease, collagen vascular disorder, diabetes mellitus and a range of other conditions.

Clinical features

In its primary form, the fingers of the upper extremities are typically affected, usually symmetrically. After exposure to cold, the fingers become cyanosed and cold. There are usually no trophic changes and fingertip necrosis is only found in unusual cases. With age, the frequency and duration of the attacks diminish. It is extremely difficult in the early phases to differentiate between primary and secondary Raynaud's disease and the additional features of collagen vascular disorders may only become apparent with the passage of time. On clinical grounds, chilblains should be differentiated from Raynaud's phenomenon. These form as a result of exposure to cold with spasm of the end arteries, leading to localized cyanosis, oedema, vesicle formation and sloughing. It is important to realize that vasospastic disorders may also be found after exposure to certain drugs, for example ergot and beta receptor blockers.

6.21.2 Functional microangiopathies

These include the following disorders: acrocyanosis occurs in young women and is due to arteriolar spasm in the capillary loops of fingers and toes. Erythrocyanosis is a reddish discoloration of the skin of the calf and ankle. It may also co-exist with acrocyanosis and usually regresses spontaneously after puberty. Erythromelalgia is paroxysmal redness of the fingers and toes accompanied by excess heat and local pain.

Functional microangiopathies should be distinguished from organic forms which include diabetic and inflammatory microangiopathies (Kimmelstiel-Wilson's disease, diabetic retinopathy, Henoch-Schoenlein purpura, thrombotic microangiopathy of the Moschcowitz type, Osler's disease, etc.).

Blood flow disorders may also be a consequence of changes in the blood, for example thrombocytosis, intravascular coagulation or erythrocyte aggregation. In cold agglutinin disease, the circulatory disorder results from exposure to cold. The cold agglutinins results in red cell agglutination with severe haemolysis. This condition may be detected by the presence of cryoglobulins which are found in a whole range of diseases, such as trypanosomiasis, viral pneumonia, infectious mononucleosis, mycoplasma pneumonia infection and in some types of lymphoma.

6.22 ANGIOLOGY (VENOUS SYSTEM)

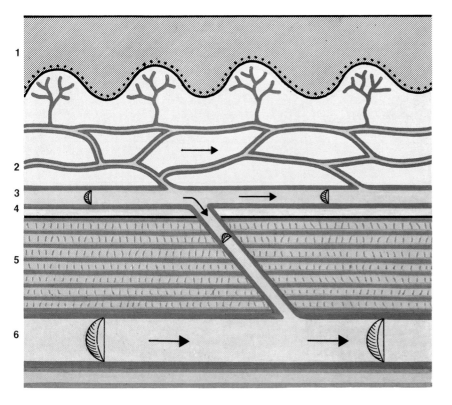

Fig. 6.112 Venous blood circulation.

1: Epidermis.
2: Subdermis.
3: Superficial vein.

4: Fascia.
5: Musculature with perforating vein.
6: Deep vein.

Fig. 6.113 Diagram of superficial and deep venous systems of the leg.

The veins are an important reservoir as they contain approximately 80% of the circulating volume of blood. This depends on the degree of constriction of the venous wall and also the venous pressure. The veins of the lungs, mesentery and legs are rich in elastic fibres, so that the blood volume can be kept constant, even with increasing venous pressure. Thin-walled veins, for example varices, will rupture even with a slight rise in pressure.

Venous pressure is determined by a range of physiological factors, for example heart rate, blood pressure, venous tone and venous flow. In the lower limbs a superficial and deep vein system is found. The deep vein system comprises the femoral vein, which collects blood from the deep veins of the calf via the popliteal veins. The superficial venous system derives its blood from the cutaneous and subcutaneous tissues of the lower limbs, and eventually, via the long saphenous vein, blood is returned to the femoral just below the inguinal ligament. The short saphenous vein drains into the popliteal vein at the back of the knee joint. There are

numerous communicating veins between the superficial and deep system. The venous system possesses valves which direct the flow of blood back to the heart. The perforating veins also have valves which ensure that blood flows from the superficial to the deep system. Venous diseases are dependent on a range of risk factors such as age, pregnancy, obesity, genetic predisposition and occupations associated with the erect posture. Other important factors include disturbance of venous flow, alteration to the venous wall and local thrombosis.

6.22.1 Varices

Definition

Varices are the result of dilatation of the vein wall and occur in various parts of the body, ranging from the pampiniform plexus (varicocele) to the oesophagus (oesophageal varices), the anus

133

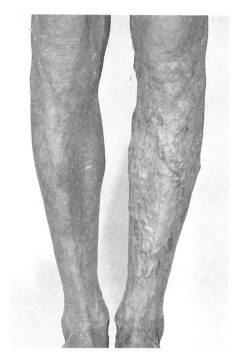

Fig. 6.114 Leg varicose veins.

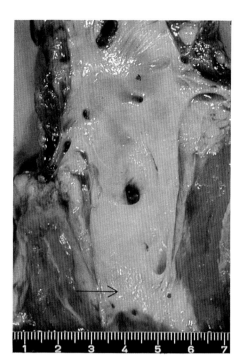

Fig. 6.115 Post phlebitic syndrome. Thickening of the intima in a varicose vein.

(haemorrhoids), the umbilicus (caput medusae) to the common varicose veins of the lower limbs (Figs 6.113 and 6.114).

Pathogenesis

A distinction should be made between primary varices, which are the common type. They occur predominantly in obese women after the age of 40 and affect the lower limbs. They are usually bilateral. They probably result from a range of pathologies. The secondary form is a result of a local cause such as thrombosis or inflammation.

Classification

1. Birch-broom varices are the mildest form. These are irregular, star-shaped, dilated veins which occur on the thighs predominantly.
2. Reticular varices. These are dilated subcutaneous veins which occur in obesity and in the elderly and may be associated with skin changes.
3. Truncal varices are irregular dilatations of the greater and lesser saphenous veins which result from abnormalities of the perforating veins with the result that the blood flow is altered and flow occurs from the deep to superficial system.

Pathology

Macroscopically, varices show evidence of venous hypertension. The intima becomes thickened and yellow and in some ways resembles arterial histology. This is particularly true in portal veins. The intima and the media become thickened with an excess of collagen fibres.

Clinical features

Initially, varicose veins of the leg are a cosmetic problem but symptoms arise later as circulation is impaired and chronic venous insufficiency occurs. A range of clinical and laboratory investigations, including the Trendelenburg test, Doppler ultrasound and phlebography, assist, in defining the problem.

Complications

About 15% of patients with varices develop superficial thrombophlebitis and, eventually, over half of the patients will develop chronic venous insufficiency. Occasionally, thrombosis may occur and occasionally the varices may rupture with extensive subcutaneous bleeding.

Trendelenburg test

Methodology
The patient lies horizontally on his back with his legs raised, allowing the blood to drain from the lower limbs. A tourniquet is then applied below the groin and is removed after the patient has stood upright for 30 seconds.

Results
(a) Negative Trendelenburg test: blood fills up slowly from below with the tourniquet still in place.
(b) Positive Trendelenburg test: despite the tourniquet, the varices fill rapidly from below upwards.
(c) Double positive Trendelenburg test: varices fill from above downwards after removal of the tourniquet. A variant of this test is Cooper's three tourniquet test.

Phlebography

In this test, the intravenous injection of contrast medium is made into a vein on the dorsum of the foot and the superficial venous system is imaged. This allows for the detection of the collateral circulation.

Doppler ultrasound

This may be of value in determining the venous flow within the varicose veins. Femoral insufficiency may be evaluated as follows:

1. Mild femoral insufficiency: retrograde venous flow may only be found during Valsalva's manoeuvre.
2. Moderate femoral insufficiency: there may be retrograde flow on deep inspiration.
3. High grade femoral insufficiency: there may be retrograde flow during normal breathing.

Venous aneurysm

This is an isolated expansion of a segment of vein. There may be a congenital or acquired valve deficiency. This is usually found in the lower limbs but may be occasionally found in the jugular vein. There is a possibility of thrombosis occurring within the abnormal segment.

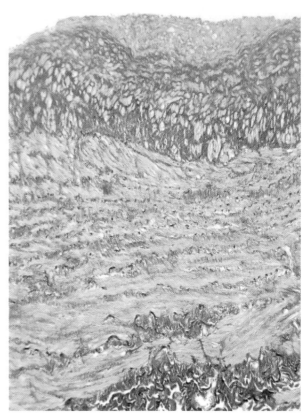

Fig. 6.116 Post phlebitic syndrome. Multiplication of collagen fibres in the intima and media of a varicose vein. van Gieson stained.

6.22.2 Thrombophlebitis and phlebothrombosis

In thrombophlebitis, the predominant features are of local inflammation in the superficial veins and this term should be restricted to disease in the superficial veins. Phlebothrombosis is thrombosis in the deep vein. Symptoms of this are present in less than 50% of patients.

The pathogenesis is that presented in 1856 by Virchow.

1. Changes in the composition of the blood (increased viscosity and hyper-coagulability)
2. Changes in the venous return
3. Changes in the vascular wall (inflammation or thrombosis)

An important precipitating factor is bed rest. Deep vein thrombosis (Fig. 6.117) frequently occurs after surgical intervention (in up to 30% of surgical patients). In the most severe cases there may be a painful purple discoloration of the limb with congestion of the superficial vein and this may proceed to venous gangrene (phlegmasia caerulia dolens).

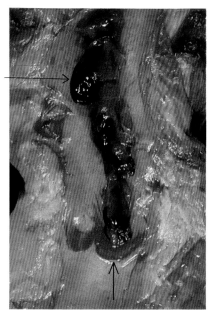
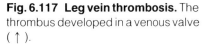

Fig. 6.117 Leg vein thrombosis. The thrombus developed in a venous valve (↑).

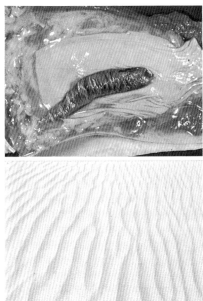

Fig. 6.118 Ribbed thrombus.

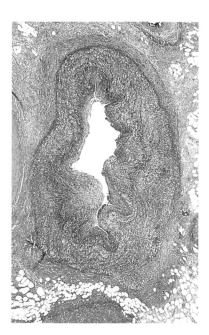

Fig. 6.119 Septic phlebitis. Diffuse leucocytic infiltration of the vein wall.

At the other extreme, many patients will only show minimal clinical signs, such as mild oedema, manifesting as an increased circumference of the limb and occasionally the earliest feature may be the onset of pulmonary embolism from a clinically inapparent deep vein thrombosis. Venous thrombosis may also arise in the pelvic veins or in association with an indwelling venous catheter. In small children with dehydration, there may be thrombosis of the inferior vena cava or the renal veins.

Thrombophlebitis migrans is one of the range of para-neoplastic syndromes and may be present in association with carcinoma of stomach, pancreas, prostate and lungs. It has also been found in association with haematological malignancies, such as leukaemia, and may be found in association with polycythaemia and rickettsial infection. In this syndrome, the clinical picture is that of a migrating thrombophlebitis in which the vein becomes painful, there is local tenderness and swelling and the overlying skin may be red. The local lesions regress quickly in a few days and reappear in another segment of superficial vein.

Pathology

In the case of venous thrombosis there is intra-vascular formation of thrombus. This usually starts at the base of a valve in an area of low flow and by accretion grows up the lumen of the vein. The thrombi lie loosely in the vascular lumen and in the course of the disease may become adherent to the vein walls. Macroscopically, the thrombi are of uniform dark colour due to incorporation of red cells. Histologically the thrombus is composed of masses of red cells bound with fibrin. Platelets and white cells are also incorporated but are usually very scanty. Differential staining of the thrombus can be performed to highlight the platelet and fibrin constituents.

Fate of the thrombus

The thrombus may detach itself to form an embolism or it may undergo spontaneous lysis. In addition, the process of organization occurs quite rapidly with the ingrowth of capillaries from the vascular wall, followed rapidly by the deposition of collagen fibres. In the final stage of organization, capillaries restore the vascular continuity (recanalization). The process of organization takes 4–6 weeks.

136

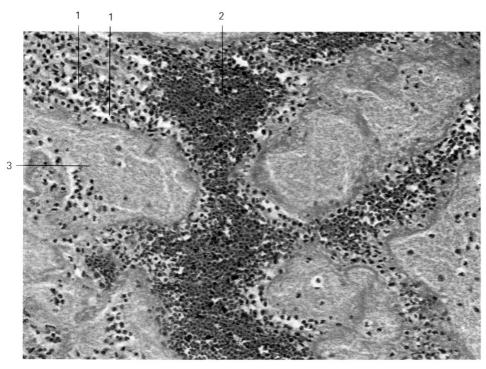

Fig. 6.120 Layered thrombus. 1: Leucocytes. 2: Erythrocytes. 3: Fibrin and platelets. HE stained.

6.22.3 Chronic venous insufficiency

This is a syndrome characterized by local oedema, the presence of small subcutaneous veins on the dorsum of the foot and ulceration usually in the medial border of the calf. There is induration of the surrounding skin, with pigmentation and an eczematous reaction. As healing occurs, thin atrophic scars appear and these easily break down to produce further ulceration.

Chronic venous insufficiency is characterized by an increase in venous pressure, distension of the veins and nutritional impairment of the surrounding skin. It is felt that a large percentage of these patients may have had previous deep vein thrombosis and, in these situations, it is best to call this the post-phlebitic syndrome.

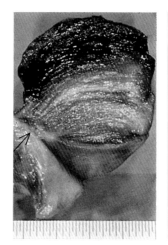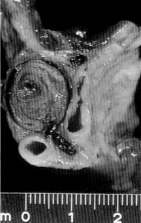

Fig. 6.121 Layered thrombi in the vein lumen. Left: thrombus already adherent to the wall (→).

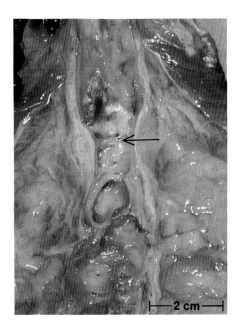

Fig. 6.122 String-of-pearls appearance (←) as an expression of old, recanalized venous thrombosis.

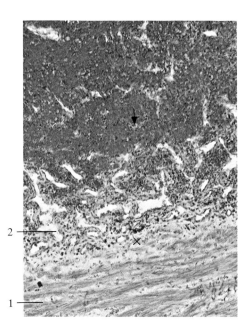

Fig. 6.123 Thrombus in the process of organization. 1: vascular media. 2: Capillaries of granulation tissue. HE stained. (↓) = fresh thrombus.

6.23 ANGIOLOGY (LYMPHATIC SYSTEM)

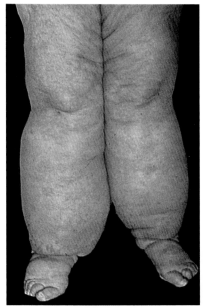

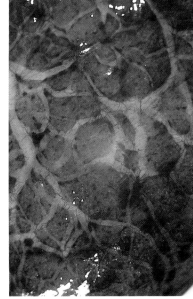

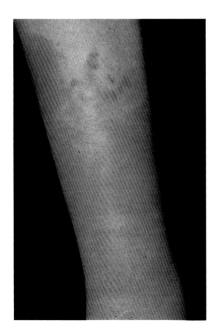

Fig. 6.124 Tropical elephantiasis.

Fig. 6.125 Scarred and obliterated subpleural lymph vessels after inflammation.

Fig. 6.126 Erysipelas.

The lymphatic system comprises the lymph vessels, lymph nodes and the thoracic duct which opens into the venous system. A lymphatic system is found only in tissues with a blood supply and is therefore absent in the cornea, the epithelium, nervous system and placenta. The lymph vessels themselves consist of three layers: the tunica interna, with endothelial cells and basement membrane; the media, with elastic and collagen fibres as well as smooth muscle fibres; and the external coat with the nerve and vaso vasorum. The lymphatic collection vessels also contain valves which are made up of three layers and contain only occasional smooth muscle cells. The lymphatic capillaries start blind-ended and form a branched, looped system with saccular expansions. They have no basement membrane and can therefore allow the passage of large molecules through the walls. The capillaries are anchored to the regional connective tissue by external anchoring filaments with collagen fibres and therefore do not collapse even in the situation of lymphoedema. Lymph flow has been termed the extravascular circulation and is regulated by capillary/tissue pressure. Pathological changes in the lymphatic system are linked to those in the cardiovascular system.

6.23.1 Lymphoedema

Lymphoedema is the lymphatic congestion caused by a primary disturbance in the lymphatic system. It is present in all forms of oedema, no matter what cause, for example cardiac, renal, etc. Distinction can be made between:

(a) Primary lymphoedema, in which there is aplasia or hypoplasia of the lymphatic vessels. The congenital form of this is called Milroy's disease.
(b) Secondary lymphoedema results from external causes, such as infections, trauma, irradiation or obstruction by carcinoma.

Severity of lymphoedema:

1. Reversible lympoedema regresses when the legs are placed horizontally
2. Irreversible oedema does not regress
3. Elephantiasis (Fig. 6.124)

6.23.2 Lymphangitis

This is inflammation of the lymph vessels indicating the spread of infection within them. It is easily

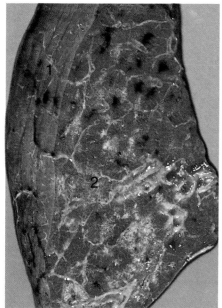
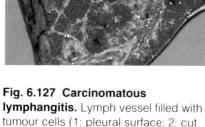
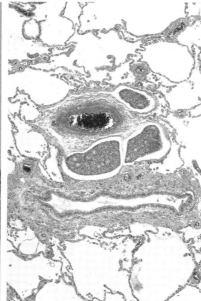
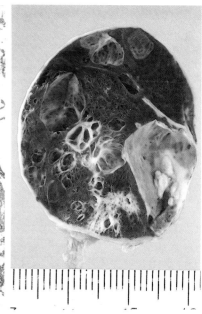

Fig. 6.127 Carcinomatous lymphangitis. Lymph vessel filled with tumour cells (1: pleural surface; 2: cut surface of the lung).

Fig. 6.128 Carcinomatous lymphangitis. A gland-forming carcinoma is present in the dilated peribronchial lymph vessels. HE stained.

Fig. 6.129 Lymphatic cysts in the spleen.

seen in the skin. The pathogenic organism, often a steptococcus, enters through small skin defects and, after an incubation period, linear red streaks appear on the skin and these spread centrally. The patient will also have high fever and rigor. The signs and symptoms settle rapidly with appropriate antibiotic therapy but recurrences do occur (habitual erysipelas (Fig. 6.126)). In the long term, fibrosis of the lymphatics may lead to local lymphoedema and on occasion extensive skin necrosis may occur.

Lymphangitis occurs in primary tuberculous infection and in other specific inflammation, for example filariasis, due to the presence of the parasite *Wucheria*. In this condition, long-term infection leads to lymphatic varices, chronic lymphatic congestion and skin oedema (elephantiasis).

6.23.3 Lymphatic cysts

These are circumscribed, uni- or multi-locular lymphangiectasia. They have to be distinguished from lymphangiomas and they secrete a clear or chylous fluid into the endothelium-lined lumen. They may be found especially in the intestinal tract, in the retroperitoneal space and in the spleen.

140

6.24 TUMOURS

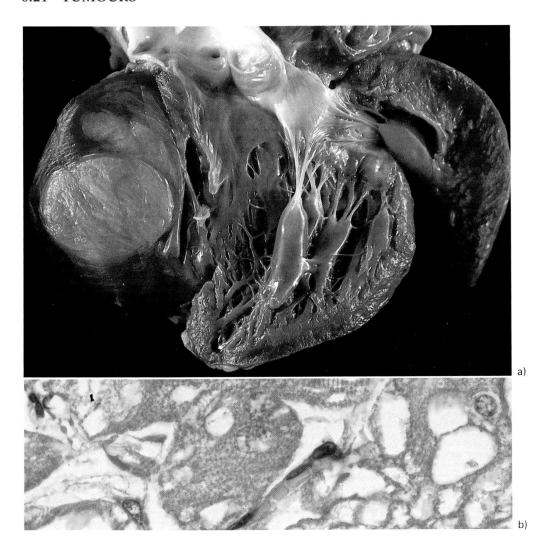

Fig. 6.130 Rhabdomyoma in the ventricular septum. b) Cross-striation and copious glycogen in the tumour cell cytoplasm. HE stained.

6.24.1 Cardiac tumours

Tumours may arise in pericardium, myocardium and endocardium and occur as a result of metastases. Primary cardiac tumours are extremely rare (0.03–0.02% on autopsy) and mainly involve atrial myxomas in adults and rhabdomyomas in children.

Rhabdomyoma

This is a primary, intracardiac lesion and, in 90% of cases, may be multiple. The aetiology is unknown but there may be associated increase in cardiac glycogen and also associated hamartoma of the conduction system. Macroscopically, there are solitary or multiple nodules which are brown in colour and located within the heart wall and occasionally in the ventricles. Histological examination shows the typical cells (arachnocytes), which are large, rounded myocytes with a cytoplasm rich in glycogen, and a central, elongated nucleus. The clinical findings are varied and include stillbirth, sudden cardiac death following arrhythmias and heart failure. Rhabdomyomas are also observed as a chance autopsy finding.

141

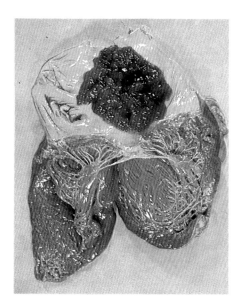

Fig. 6.131 Cardiac myxoma. Papillary growth in the left atrium, adherent to the wall.

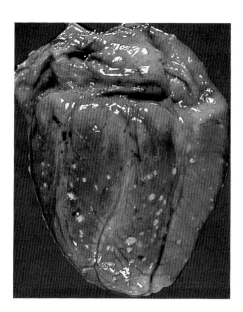

Fig. 6.132 Multiple subendocardial metastases of a bronchial carcinoma.

Cardiac myxoma

This is usually a solitary, pedunculated neoplasm which may grow up to 6cm in diameter. It is often located within the left atrium (70% of cases) and is frequently found in women between 30 and 60 years of age. It is neoplastic in origin and is thought to arise from the endothelial cell layer. Histologically, it is rich in mucopolysaccharides and contains stellate myxomatous cells rich in haemosiderin in the stoma, with fibrinous deposits at the periphery. Myxoma presents clinically due to local circulatory disturbance (i.e. deficient atrial filling, blockage of the mitral orifice), or by the production of distant emboli with multiple peripheral infarctions.

Papillary fibroelastoma

These occur in the region of the heart valves and may also be known as papillary heart valve tumours (Lambl's excrescence). The growths usually arise in adulthood and affect the aortic valve and more rarely the parietal endocardium. Macroscopically, it consists of a rich network of delicately branched collagen fibres covered with loose connective tissue and elastic fibres. The clinical presentation is nonspecific.

Fibroma of the heart

This tumour arises in the ventricular septum in infants and children. Macroscopically, it has well-defined white, firm nodules. These are histologically composed of collagen and elastic fibres with occasional smooth muscle cells. These slow-growing tumours give rise to arrhythmias due to compression of the conduction system.

Pericardial mesothelioma

This neoplasm corresponds morphologically to pleural mesothelioma. However, there seem to be no causal associations with asbestosis. The tumour spreads over the heart surface and penetrates the superficial layers of the myocardium. It is frequently accompanied by a pericardial effusion, which produces clinical symptoms. Other rare primary malignant tumours of the heart include rhabdomyosarcoma, angiosarcoma and mesothelioma of the conducting system.

Cardiac metastases

The heart is rarely a site for secondary neoplasia. They may arise as a result of the spread of a neighbouring primary tumour (bronchial or oesophageal). Haematogenous metastases may occur from malignant melanoma, breast and kidney carcinomas. Lymphomatoid or leukaemic infiltrations may also occur. The clinical presentation is determined by the primary tumour and the cardiac manifestations depend on the part of the heart which is infiltrated.

6.24.2 Vascular tumours

Vascular tumours have a broad spectrum of presentation. They may appear in the vessel wall and are themselves very vascular, being composed of multitudinous growing vessels. Benign vascular tumours (haemangiomas) are frequently indistinguishable from hamartomas. Vascular tumours tend to grow until puberty and then may regress spontaneously. They may, on occasion, be malignant. The common sites are skin, nervous system, liver and spleen. They may be identified immunohistochemically because of the presence of factor VIII antigen, a reflection of their endothelial content.

Classification of the major vascular tumours:

I. Histological classification.
1. Tumours of the vascular wall:
   Leiomyoma   Leiomyosarcoma
2. Tumours of the vessels:
   1. Blood vessels:
      Haemangioendothelioma   Haemangio-
                               endothelio-
                               sarcoma

      Capillary haemangioma
      Cavernous haemangioma
      Venous haemangioma
      Glomus tumour   Malignant
                               glomus
                               tumour

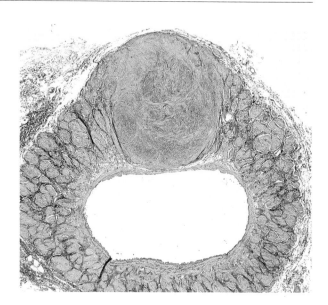

Fig. 6.133 Leiomyoma in the wall of a renal vein. van Gieson stained.

Capillary haemangiomas

These occur mainly in young children and are commonly present at birth. The main place affected is the face but other organs may also be involved, particularly the central nervous system. Macroscopically, they are highly vascular tumours. They

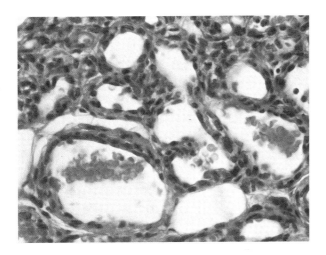

Fig. 6.134 Capillary haemangioma. HE stained.

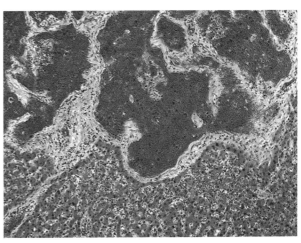

Fig. 6.135 Cavernous haemangioma of the liver. HE stained.

may be slightly raised above the skin surface and have a sharp margin (Fig. 6.134). Histologically, the tumour is composed of a solid endothelium with capillary differentiation. Mitoses occur occasionally and atypical cells are absent. The growth has no capsule and there is no infiltration. Myohaemangioma is a separate disease which has to be distinguished from sarcoma by its frequent mitoses.

Cavernous haemangiomas

These occur in the skin of the face, trunk and limbs and may be a chance finding in the liver at laparotomy or autopsy. These liver haemangiomas may be picked up routinely on CT scanning or ultrasound of the liver. The lesions remain asymptomatic and become scarred and fibrotic with age as local thrombosis occurs (Fig. 6.135). They may occasionally bleed if traumatized.

Venous haemangioma

This is a new growth occurring mainly in the skin and composed of various sizes of irregularly arranged veins. A variant, which contains looped arteries, may be found in the brain and meninges (Ranke's haemangioma).

Eruptive haemangioma

This consists of leashes of overgrown capillaries on the skin of the fingers or the mucosa of the lips. It has an epidermal covering.

Haemangiomatosis

This is a condition in which multiple flat haemangioma are found in multiple organs. A range of clinical syndromes have been described:

1. Bean's syndrome: skin and intestinal haemangiomatosis
2. De Bailey's syndrome: kidney
3. Louis-Bar's syndrome: telangiectasis and ataxia
4. Hippel-Lindau's syndrome: CNS and ocular haemangioma
5. Sturge-Weber's syndrome: broad, flat facial naevus with meningeal involvement
6. Klippel-Trenaunay's syndrome: limb naevus with local giantism
7. Rendu-Osler's syndrome: telangiectasis of the skin, liver, lungs and CNS.

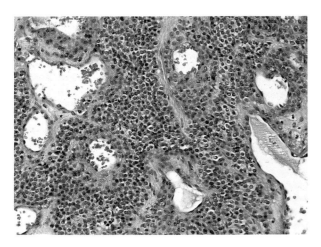

Fig. 6.136 Glomus tumour. HE stained.

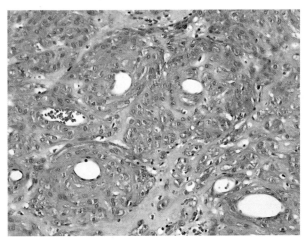

Fig. 6.137 Angiomyoma (vascular leiomyoma).
van Gieson stained.

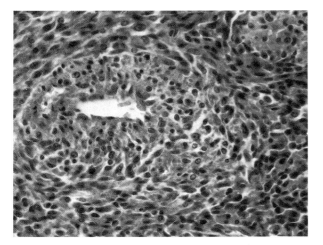

Fig. 6.138 Haemangiopericytoma. Stained for lattice
fibres.

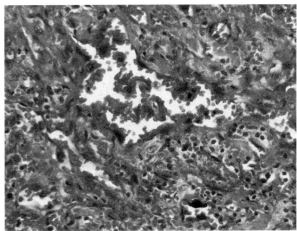

Fig. 6.139 Malignant haemangioendothelioma. HE
stained.

Glomus tumour

This arises from the glomus cells and occurs in all
organs of the body but has a preference for the
fingers (Fig. 6.136). Histologically, it consists of
large blood vessels surrounded by small cells with
round nuclei. There is angiomatous variant (vascular leiomyoma) and this is composed of con-
centrically layered smooth muscle fibres around
small blood vessels. This is commonly found in the
skin of the thigh.

Haemangiopericytoma

This is a benign tumour found in soft tissues and is
derived from pericytes (Fig. 6.138). It consists of
round, spindle-shaped cells within a dense fibrous

network. The malignant variety is difficult to distinguish histologically from the benign.

Malignant haemangioendothelioma and angiosarcoma

These are both highly malignant and occur in the
skin, liver, thyroid, spleen and lymph nodes (Fig.
6.139). Haemangioendotheliomas of liver have
been described as a result of exposure to arsenic,
Thorotrast and polyvinylchloride. These are friable
tumours and highly likely to bleed. Histologically,
they consist of densely packed endothelial cells.
The clinical features are those of a highly malignant
soft tissue sarcoma, the prognosis of which depends on the extent and degree of differentiation of
the cells.

6.24.3 Tumours of the lymphatic system

Lymphangiomas

These are benign tumours composed of lymphatic vessels with normal endothelium (Fig. 6.140). They occur in the head, chest, neck and limbs of children and the following forms are histologically distinguishable.

1. Capillary lymphangioma: this has a highly proliferative, although not atypical, endothelium. Differentiation from capillary haemangiomas is difficult.
2. Cavernous haemangioma show broad cavities lined by endothelium containing an amorphous, slightly acidophilic mass.
3. Cystic lymphangioma (hygromas): these are soft, diffuse, painless swellings in the lateral parts of the neck and occasionally in the axillary cavity. They are often detectable at birth.

Lymphangiomyoma

This is a variant of cavernous lymphangioma, with numerous smooth muscle cells. It is found usually in women in the thoracic duct and it may lead to recurrent chylothorax. When an entire region of the body is affected, it is called lymphangiomyomatosis.

Lymphangiosarcoma (malignant lymphangioendothelioma)

This is a malignant tumour composed of irregularly arranged lymph vessels with greatly thickened atypical endothelium (Figs 6.141–6.142). This is a rare type of sarcoma which develops in skin previously involved with chronic lymphoedema. A variant is the Stewart-Treves syndrome in which lymphangiosarcoma may form in an area of skin previously involved from previous mastectomy and lymphadenectomy.

Kaposi's sarcoma

This is a tumour of unknown origin which behaves as an angiosarcoma. This tumour is now found extensively in Africa, where it comprises 9% of all malignant tumours in Uganda and is now recognized to be a complication of HIV infection. Kaposi's sarcoma mainly affects the skin, although it is found in internal organs. Multiple brown-red purple nodules are seen macroscopically and histological examination reveals an angiomatous capillary component and a solid spindle-cell one. The prognosis is poor and rapidly leads to death.

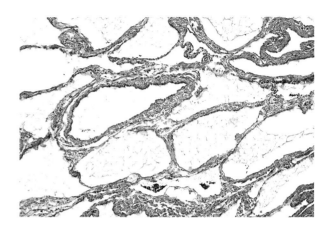

Fig. 6.140 **Lymphangioma.** van Gieson stained.

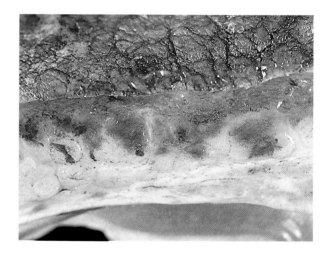

Fig. 6.141 **Lymphangiosarcoma** of the skin associated with chronic oedema (Stewart-Treves' syndrome).

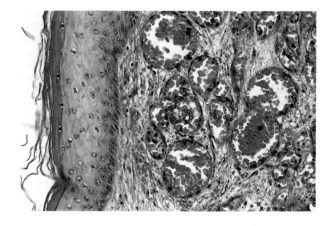

Fig. 6.142 **Lymphangiosarcoma.** HE stained.

Index

Page numbers in *italic* refer to figures